Chair Yoga & Wall Pilates For Seniors

Enhance Your Flexibility & Posture, Improve Balance & Independence, Alleviate Pain and Lose Weight under 10 mins a day

Chair Yoga for Seniors

Quick and Effective Wall Pilates for Seniors

Laurel Harris

CONTENTS

Chair Yoga for Seniors
153 Easy Poses for Weight Loss, Pain Relief, Balance, & Independence

Quick and Effective Wall Pilates for Seniors
50+ Easy Step-by-Step Poses, to Improve Balance, Alleviate Pain, Strengthen the Core, to Enhance Flexibility & Posture in Under 10 Minutes a Day.

CHAIR YOGA FOR SENIORS

153 Easy Poses for Weight Loss, Pain Relief, Balance, & Independence

LAUREL HARRIS

Introduction

Reclaim Your Vitality, Redefine Your Golden Years with Chair Yoga

A few years ago, I was in my mid-sixties, and boy, was I feeling it. The slight aches and pains from my fifties had become permanent participants in my daily life. I suffered from a different type of exhaustion, a non-physical kind that only people who are older can understand. I was living well, doing my best to maximize my time by doing what I enjoy, engaging with family, etc., and even working to take care of my body by walking every day. Yet, while life was good, and I enjoyed my time with my family, I always knew deep down that it could be better.

Without using hyperbole, half an hour of exercise for a week was enough to change my life. I was asked by a more youthful friend to join her in some yoga, which I agreed to, but due to my reduced mobility, I had to carry out the exercises while seated. I woke up the next day, and the permanent aches were a little less pronounced. I practiced the yoga again the next day, and lo and behold, the pain lessened even more.

Realizing the connection between exercise and my wellness, I invested some time and effort into looking for ways to maximise the effect while accommodating my age and limited ability. That's how I came across Chair Yoga, and within a few weeks, I felt like a completely new person. I was able to move better, which doesn't sound like a lot but is revolutionary.

That's the summary of my story, and it could be yours too. The many benefits of yoga are self-evident as soon as you get started. Increasing flexibility, improving balance and posture, alleviating/relieving aches and pains, better physical and emotional health, an increase in energy levels, potential for turning the activity into a social one as well by joining yoga groups, as well as a feeling of independence and taking charge. Something not everybody mentions is that by maintaining your mobility, you gain independence. There is no need to have people always around to do things for you since you can do them yourself. Something that feels obvious yet can make a world of difference, whether it's chasing after grandchildren or cleaning the house and taking out the trash.

A useful statistic to give some perspective on the matter at hand: "More than one-third of persons 65 years of age or older fall each year, and in half of such cases, the falls are recurrent. The risk doubles or triples in the presence of cognitive impairment or a history of previous falls. In Canada, falls are the most common cause (85%) of injury-related hospital admissions among those aged 65 years or older" (Al-Aama, 2011).

In this book, the goal will be to answer three of the most practical and impactful questions regarding chair yoga, especially for those over 60: What does chair yoga actually entail (including some significant differences between it and other forms of yoga)? What does it actually do for you/what are the benefits? What makes it better than other alternatives/what makes it the best choice of activity?

Without over-explaining the methodology, we will further explore in this book that there is a unique approach to the implementation of it you will get from this book. To maximise the effectiveness of your chair yoga exercises, I have incorporated the "SENIOR FRAMEWORK" into the book. There are multiple "levels" where your exercises can be better tailored to your overall ability and fitness levels. You can then work through the levels and increase the difficulty and complexity of the exercises as you desire.

Not only are the benefits profound and widespread when you practice chair yoga but paired with the "SENIOR FRAMEWORK" and using the exercises I will outline in this book, you can experience the results so much faster than ever before. While it won't occur suddenly, noticeable effects could emerge within a few days; you may already begin to feel them. The timeline for observing changes may vary, especially for those who are overweight, less physically active, or dealing with health conditions. Upon waking in the morning, you should experience a sense of invigoration, refreshment, and a lack of aches. To the extent that you might even find yourself rejuve- nated enough to spontaneously join in activities like playing soccer with your grandkid's kids.

I was in a situation where I needed the benefits of chair yoga, and I found them. I then spent a few years learning and mastering the available techniques and movements. I have pulled together over 150 of the most beneficial exercises, ranging in difficulty and complexity, that I will include in this book. Paired with the SENIOR FRAMEWORK to assist in progression through the exercises. You can become the life of the party again, and all of this is achieved without hours of backbreaking work. Simply from the comfort of your own chair, you can change the course of your life and do as we all desire. Age With Grace.

CHAPTER 1

WHY CHOOSE CHAIR YOGA?

Does growing old cause you to become inactive, or does inactivity cause you to grow old?

As an older citizen, exercising regularly is arguably one of the most important actions you can carry out to improve your health. It can do a lot to delay or even prevent some health problems and minimize the physical deterioration you might experience as you age.

According to a study published in the journal Circulation, exercising more than 300 minutes per week if it is an intense workout or 600 minutes for a light workout (about two hours of activity daily, inclusive of walking five days a week) can reduce risk of mortality by 31% (*Exercising More Than Recommended Could Lengthen Life, Study Suggests*, 2022). From a holistic point of view, aerobics is the best form of adult exercise. It manages to combine all the essential physical aspects that exercise engages into one long-form workout type.

The benefits of exercise are numerous. The most profound benefit is the mental health benefit since exercising regularly reduces stress and anxiety by regulating the brain neurotransmitters that control stress levels, among others. It also aids in the release of endorphins that improve your mood and allow you to sleep better. Exercising regularly also brings some much needed repetition into your life as a senior. Due to retirement, life can be a little unstructured and chaotic otherwise. As a bonus, you also become stronger and feel more capable and secure. In the brain, exercise helps keep the brain functions harmonised, which improves memory and overall cognitive ability, while if done in a group, it also creates additional social bonds, which suppresses loneliness.

Exercising strengthens muscles and strengthens the bones as well. It stimulates and promotes the maintenance of bone strength, density, and cellular regeneration. Exercises that focus on balance and flexibility also assist by reducing the likelihood of falls, which are the biggest cause of fractures and broken bones, especially in seniors.

COMMON BARRIERS TO EXERCISE FOR SENIORS

While reasons for not exercising can be numerous, there are usually many ways to work around it effectively. The main reasons people don't/can not exercise are listed below.

Physical Limitations - The cause of a physical inability to exercise might be chronic illness, chronic pain, and disability. These aren't scenarios that can be changed easily, yet with some thought and determination, you can overcome these or work around them.

Lack of Motivation - Whether it's simply not caring, a lack of confidence, believing oneself incapable, or fear of injury. At times, older adults lack the necessary motivation to carry out the arduous work of exercising regularly.

Accessibility Issues - The cost of gym memberships, costs of exercise implements, and, depending on your location, the presence of gyms in general can all cause people not to exercise.

Lack of Time - Some seniors continue to work highly demanding jobs and take care of their families, both of which take up a lot of time and energy, and so being the higher priority, the adult does not make time or, worse, cannot find time to exercise at all.

Social Isolation - Exercising in a group encourages and motivates those engaging in it. Whereas if you exercise alone, you are more likely to miss days or give up. Worse yet, as older adults, if they exercise with their partner when that partner passes, they might cease exercising altogether.

Depression - Overall, depression lessens the individual's desire to carry out any activity. In older adults, such a condition is common due to the loss of friends and partners and usually declining mental health. This means they can be less motivated and willing to exercise.

How Exercise Affects Independence

Enhanced Mobility - The exercise helps/maintain muscle strength and joint flexibility, which in turn helps seniors maintain their full range of motion. The exercise also promotes stability and coordination, which ensures users maintain fine motor control of their body, with some flexibility training even enhancing their comfortable range of movement.

Reduced Risk of Falling - With exercises that promote strength, stability, general coordination, and balance, you are a lot less likely to fall over due to the muscular degeneration and loss of coordination that would otherwise occur as you age.

Boosting Self-Confidence - Exercising in a group significantly boosts social ties and engagement. This prevents those involved from feeling lonely or, worse yet, suffering from significant bouts of depression.

CHAIR YOGA IS THE BEST CHOICE FOR SENIORS

Low-Risk High Reward

In general, chair yoga encompasses all of the already mentioned. It strengthens you; it enhances coordination, balance, and stability. It reduces joint pain, has mental health benefits, and more.

To add to that, it is also one of the safest exercises for seniors. It does not require significant weight, it does not put a lot of strain on the body, and it is easy on the joints and muscles, which is good for those with arthritis or hampered mobility. It is an aerobic exercise and so improves/manages circulation, providing cardio-vascular benefits. You gain a decent bit of flexibility from yoga exercises since they require stretching. With that comes increased balance and coordination and reduced stress. It is also known that yoga can reduce the aches and pains that seniors often suffer from.

Access and Convenience

Another benefit of Chair Yoga is that it is really easy to get into. The barrier to entry into it is really low since there is no need for any complex equipment apart from a comfortable and sturdy chair you can use, meaning there is zero cost attached to it. The exercises can be done from anywhere and are suited to those with limited mobility. Many of the exercises can also be tweaked to make them achievable for people with any disabilities as well.

Holistic Health Benefits

Overall gains from the exercise benefit the entire person. Yoga brings some unity between the body and the mind, relieving stress and increasing self-confidence. There is also the production of positive brain chemicals which improve sleep and reduce anxiety/depression. As an additional benefit, yoga also gives you better posture and overall balance, which prevents you from developing a hunched neck and back.

How often should you engage in it? - For the most part, exercising two to three times a week is the minimum, and stepping up the amount provides greater benefits. Long-term commitment is recommended, but as a beginner, even one to two weekly sessions are a great start.

Precautions

Make sure to speak to your doctor before engaging in the physical activity aspect. Just in case, there is a consideration you must make when exercising. Additionally, do not overexert yourself; know your limitations and respect them, especially if you have not been working out before this. Additionally, your body communicates with you. Listen to what it is saying: If you feel exhausted, stop; if you feel significant pain, stop!

By now, you should have an answer to the question - Does growing old cause you to become inactive, or does inactivity cause you to grow old?

In the next chapter, we have a high-level discussion of the science behind chair yoga, validating its merits with some hard data.

CHAPTER 2

THE SCIENCE BEHIND THE CHAIR

Science doesn't lie; chair yoga is more than just stretching and controlled breathing, and the benefits go beyond just that, too. Research and data is coming out daily that challenge what we know and what we think we know about most things. In the realm of senior health and well-being, the reality that yoga, and in this specific case chair yoga, has never been challenged by the found data; instead, it has been fully reinforced at every opportunity.

ANATOMY OF A YOGA POSE

Part of the research carried out has found that different specific muscle groups are engaged when different yoga poses are engaged. The maximum benefits are for those who achieve skill mastery since they can achieve better muscular utilisation during each pose, which should serve to inspire beginners to take on the challenge.

Understanding Muscle Engagement

Muscle alignment is the term given to the absolute, perfectly precise way to enter into and hold a yoga pose in the way most beneficial to you while also providing the least risk of injury. Alignment isn't a fixed state; however, bodies are different, and their capabilities vary considerably. The concept is instead based on fulfilling the requirements of a pose, engaging those muscle groups to actually see the benefits. You can make use of props and chairs to achieve this.

Importance of Alignment

Alignment is important as it prevents any long-term yoga injuries (that are very rare) from repeated, misaligned poses that might harm you. It also looks to ensure that you are in as optimal a position as you can achieve in order to maximise your poses.

Breath Control

Yoga and breathing are intrinsically connected. Without breath management, yoga is significantly less effective and potentially harmful. All interested parties must learn when to inhale and when to exhale. The five rules of breathing are listed below.

1. **Inhale When Opening the Front of The Body** - When raising the arms and spreading them outward, raising the head, bending backward, etc. When you push your chest out, always inhale.

2. **Exhale When Compressing the Front of the Body** - when you move the chest inward or forward, you compress the lungs and diaphragm. Therefore, in all forward bends, twists, and side bends (touch your toes), be sure always to exhale.

3. **If Post Inhalation Breath Is Suspended, Do Not Move** - When you reach the maximum point of inhalation (lungs are filled - chest is fully expanded). At that point, you can hold the breath to extend the inhalation, but if/when doing so, do not move; if you decide to move, do not hold the breath at all; let it out immediately.

4. **Only Move During Breath Suspension if it's Following an Exhalation.** Exhalations can be extended by holding your breath post-exhalation. In this case, you can move during the held breath.

5. Breathe Deeply and Effortlessly - In any situation where breathing is strained, it is a sign you have pushed too far. Yoga should be comfortable; breathing should be naturally deep, not forced or hurried, and should be without strain or disruption. Do not strain the body.

However, don't worry too much; you do not need to memorise all this; simply implement it slowly over time.

How Does it Result in Physiological Benefits?

How it Aids Weight Loss

Yoga is physical exercise and so burns calories as you carry it out. It also reduces stress, stress which causes an increase in the hormone cortisol, which in turn increases abdominal fat, decreases muscle and causes sugar cravings. It can also help overcome negative eating behaviours by mitigating stress and anxiety. (Mph, 2021)

Pain Relief Mechanisms

Yoga moves the body in harmony. Controlled breathing, physical movement, and meditation can result in a good alignment of the body's components. Benefits include lessened migraines, decreased chronic pain, fibromyalgia, low back pain, and so on (Harvard Health, 2015).

Improving Balance and Coordination

The intentional movements of yoga require your muscle groups to adapt to be able to hold a pose for as long as is required. You often see yoga practitioners who are able to remain balanced while holding a pose for over 2 minutes. This means the muscles in the body are trained to maintain stability and balance while eliminating unwanted twitches and movements, which boosts coordination.

Stress Reduction

I have already mentioned that exercising can reduce stress, but now it's time to look at the specific science of how that is possible. Yoga involves stretching the muscles, which in turn relieves muscle tension that builds up from stress. It also activates the parasympathetic nervous system, which reduces stress. Yoga exercises oppose the negative effects of stress; they reduce blood pressure and heart rate while improving the efficiency of respiration. It encourages awareness, which decreases worrying and stress. The peacefulness of the exercise also permits one to have a mental break, which is simply time spent with a clear mind, without stress or worry.

Cognitive Improvements

For an aging mind, care should be taken to keep it engaged in healthy and beneficial activities. This helps put off the onset of conditions such as dementia, memory loss, and general mental degradation. Yoga requires a calm focus and intensity to hold poses well; this improves/maintains the practitioner's ability to concentrate and focus for extended periods. It also improves the attention span of those partaking.

The learning process for the many different poses and breathing techniques provides stimulus for the brain's memory centres, which helps keep the mind sharp and able to recall things better. The poses engage the motor skills, which guarantees the maintenance, if not improvement, of motor skills, as well as the acquisition of all new and finer motor skills. The physical side of exercise also sees increased blood flow and respiratory efficiency, which means more oxygen delivery to the brain. The additional stress relief and promoted balance also play a role in ensuring the brain is as protected from age-based decline as possible.

Emotional Well Being

Yoga brings about a state of relaxation and calm in users, which does away with stress and anxiety. A more significant benefit is it can help overcome depression and improve the quality of sleep. Getting a healthy amount of rest every night is an important factor in mental and emotional health and stability.

The physical exercise aspect means retained mobility and independence, which help seniors feel more in control of their lives and their bodies. You also become more in tune with your body, which helps you understand and accept what it is capable of, and understand your limitations and your capabilities. Yoga is a very social activity, which means it plays a role in reducing loneliness and isolation.

There is a lot of data and research that has backed up the impact and efficacy of chair yoga in improving the lives of seniors. That, on its own, should be enough of an incentive to look into how to start incorporating it into your daily life as quickly as possible. In the next chapter, we will look at just that. How to get started with chair yoga, the physical and emotional preparation, as well as the equipment needed.

CHAPTER 3

GETTING STARTED WITH CHAIR YOGA: WHAT YOU NEED

Getting started with chair yoga is easier than putting on a pair of shoes, and honestly, you don't even need shoes. When I said the barrier to entry is essentially non-existent, I meant it. You can make do with just about any chair in your home. However, to optimize your environment for chair yoga, here are some pointers.

CHOOSING THE RIGHT CHAIR

There are some basic areas to look into when selecting a chair for chair yoga. The main points of consideration are listed and explained below:

1. **Physical Layout** - The seating surface of the chair must be flat and a little hard. This means no camping chairs that sag in the middle, no sofas, and so forth. Rather, find a chair with a sturdy seat base and material. Additionally, the chair cannot have armrests on either side; they will limit your range of motion and make some poses a lot more challenging or unachievable entirely.

The chair height should be such that your feet can rest flat on the ground with your knees at a solid 90 degrees while sitting comfortably. If the chair has height adjustability, padding on the seat, and a backrest that increases comfort without disrupting the necessary flatness while sitting, then that's even better.

2. **Stability** - The chair you select should not be wobbly or tip over very easily. It should have a wide and solid base that ensures it has maximum weight distribution and stability. Avoid chairs with wheels as well; they reduce the overall stability of the chair; some yoga poses leverage the chair to support you and might result in injury if the chair were to roll out while you are using it to keep you upright. Use rubber non-slip end caps for your chairs, or place the chair on a yoga mat to prevent slipping or, worse yet, potentially scuffing/scratching your floors.

3. **Comfort and Usability** - While you should want the chair to be comfortable and not assault your backside, the main priority should remain to find a chair that is stable first and foremost. If you can get a hold of a chair that has a backrest that can lean/bend backward or even one that has a removable backrest, then that's even better. Since that gives you added flexibility in how you can move and pose, it may also incentivise trying some more challenging poses when you are at an advanced level.

Overall, most chairs around the homework well enough; regular kitchen or dining table chairs work fine (chairs and not stools or sofas), given they are not too high vertically and they have a wide and stable base. Office chairs work fine as well; if the armrests are removable, then go for it. Regardless, though, most chairs that fulfil the above-listed requirements will work fine. You can even buy specialised yoga chairs, but it's not a requirement.

Setting up Your Space

It is usually best practice to find a dedicated space for practising chair yoga. It can be in your home, the backyard/park, or in a gym/facility somewhere. If you wish to do it in your home, but space is limited, you can move furniture around to set up your exercise space and then move it back afterwards; you will have to repeat this process daily, though. Regardless, there are a few boxes that the space you wind up selecting is expected to tick to be the optimum space for practising chair yoga.

These boxes that need ticking are:

A well-lit space, usually if natural light is available, is the most ideal, but if not, artificial light works just as well. However, make sure it is not too bright; you can use dimmers to control that.

In a cool space, the temperature has to be comfortable enough to facilitate physical activity without worry of heat exhaustion, heat stroke, etc. Usually, 70-75 degrees Fahrenheit or 21 - 24 degrees Celsius is the most ideal.

Good ventilation and fresh air must be available, and the space must not contain any strong odours.

A clean and clutter-free space, with no objects that can injure you, should be in the vicinity.

Some optional elements are:

Soft and calming music or ambient sounds at a low background volume.

If it's a group session, leave enough space between chairs to move freely.

If it's a group session, it is recommended to either arrange chairs in a circle or, if in rows then stagger the rows.

You will also find some great use for the following optional props.

Blankets, Cushions/pillows, Yoga mats, Blocks, Elastic bands (you could use a scarf or a belt if you don't have an elastic band)

What to Wear

For the most part, there isn't a specific dress code for yoga. What you want is clothing that is reasonably loose and breathable. Whatever you choose is fine unless it's so heavy that it restricts motion. Items like denim aren't recommended, and neither are heavy jackets unless the climate demands it. There is no need for yoga-specific clothing, no need to splurge money on yoga pants or shirts.

On your feet, you don't need anything. The recommendation is to go barefoot and let the dogs out. Either that or non-slip grippy socks; regular socks are too slippery and can cause injury. There are a few additional accessories, such as yoga gloves, yoga straps, and so on, which can be of some use and provide support but are not necessarily needed.

Safety Precautions

The most essential precaution is not to push beyond your limits; if you feel strain or pain, ease up. Additional precautions for safe practice include customisation/modification of poses to account for your own limitations (if you have a bad knee, etc.). Do not move too quickly or rush poses; move slowly and deliberately. Make sure you prioritise alignment as much as possible and keep a stable base for every exercise. Before going too far into poses, warm up properly, and when exercising, keep a phone close to you in case of injury or emergency.

Precautions For People With Medical Conditions

Some poses will need to be avoided or heavily changed if you have an injury/condition. We will go into this in a later chapter. This applies especially to those with hip/knee replacements or problems if you have spinal problems, osteoporosis, vertigo, and many other conditions.

Now you know all the basics needed to get started with actually practising chair yoga, are you excited to get started? In the next chapter, you will get into the business end of the book and actually start learning yoga poses.

CHAPTER 4

CHAIR YOGA FUNDAMENTALS

A home's foundation is what keeps it standing. In chair yoga, mastery of the foundational poses and breathing techniques will keep you strong and flexible as you progress through more advanced or modified exercises. In this chapter, we will look at eight fundamental poses, some breathing exercises, and a meditation pose for overall wellness.

BASIC POSES AND THEIR VARIATIONS

Here are a few foundational yoga poses and some variations for them. These poses will be an initial basis for all your early-stage yoga progress. As you take on these poses, keep the foundational elements we discussed in mind, focus on alignment, be sure to monitor your breathing, and make sure your environment is suited to the work that you are looking to do.

Yoga Flow - Yoga flow is a practice in which each pose seamlessly transitions into the next, creating a continuous and fluid sequence.

Seated Mountain Pose - Sit on a chair with your back straight and your feet firmly planted on the floor - shoulder width apart, rest your palms flat on your thighs.

Then, take a deep breath, extending your spine while simultaneously pushing your feet onto the floor (inhaling). Then, as you start to exhale, draw your stomach in and allow your shoulders to slump a little.

As you progress, include turning your head to the left or right as you inhale to give the back muscles more of a stretch.

You can then repeat this exercise as many times as you need while being sure not to overextend yourself. You should feel the back, core, and thigh muscles engaged in this use case.

If you have limited mobility, you can use the back of the chair as a support for your back and neck. If your chair has no backrest, you can prop it up against the wall for that support. Hold onto your chair and/or onto your things for support if you need it.

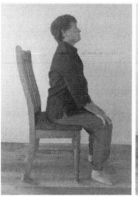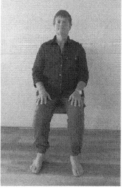

Chair Cat-Cow Stretch - Sit upright in your chair with your back straight. Then, place your palms on your thighs. You want to let your midsection lean back, pushing the hips and curving the back into a bit of a hunch.

Try to keep your head and shoulders in their initial position (just lowered) while the midsection curls backward, and you push your chest inward (inhaling).

Then, come forward, push your chest out, and tilt your head up, arching the back inward toward the thighs and knees (exhaling).

When you reach the maximum comfortable stretch on each inward/outward stretch, hold the pose for a little while, then release and slowly engage the other position.

Repeat 5-10 times, coordinating the movement with your breath.

If you have limited movement, some modifications are to arch your back less if doing so is a challenge for you. You can also use the chair for stability as you do the exercise and only move through the pose for as much as and as far as is comfortable.

Seated Forward Bend - To maximize this pose, start yourself off in the already explained seated mountain pose. Back straight, head elevated, feet pushing into the ground.

Inhaling into the seated mountain, you then breathe out as you lean forward over your thighs.

In this pose, keep your arms at your sides if you can (keep them on your knees and then lower them to your shins if you need them to support you.)

Bend as far forward as you can without pain and hold that position for a few seconds, breathing deeply before coming back to the normal position in the upright seated mountain.

Hold for 5-10 breaths.

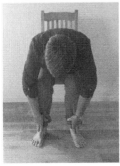 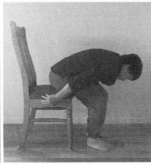 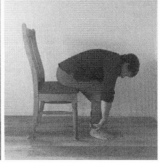

If mobility is limited, you can use a strap tied around your feet to keep the legs extended, especially if hamstring movement is limited. You can also place a rolled-up towel under your thighs to support them if the chair is not comfortable. Do not stretch your back further than is comfortable.

Breathing Techniques

Yoga (Yogic) breathing is a specific practice of breathing during yoga. If it hasn't made itself apparent at this point already, the breathing aspect is a crucial part of yoga, to the point where a lot of the exercises and poses are either less effective or ineffective if the necessary breathing does not accompany the pose.

The benefits of this breathing are that it is calming and reduces stress, but it also ensures our body functions are regulated as we exercise. Breathing ensures our muscles and brain get the required oxygen, keeps our blood pressure and heart rate in check, and activates the parasympathetic nervous system. Additionally, breathing increases lung capacity in the yoga practitioner. Overall, better well-being is experienced by all who engage in yogic breathing. Here are a few breathing exercises:

Diaphragmatic Breathing - This is a breathing practice that requires you to be seated. Place one hand on the belly button region and the other on the lower ribs. Breathe from the diaphragm; you should feel your hands rising. Do it for multiple minutes - up to about 10 should be fine. To ensure you are doing it accurately, the hand on your belly button should rise before the one on your ribs; that's how you confirm you're doing it right.

Alternate Nostril Breathing - Rest your left hand on your thigh and your right on your face. Then go ahead and hold the right nostril closed with the thumb and breathe in through the left nostril only. Alternate to the other nostril with the other hand and then exhale with the right nostril. Inhale with the right nostril and breathe out with the left. Continue this process of alternating nostrils for 5 minutes; this calms the mind.

Ocean Breath - This is a simple one. Inhale very deeply, keeping your mouth closed. Bring the tongue to the roof of your mouth. Then you exhale through the nose again - mouth still closed and constrict the throat muscles as you do this. In theory, it should sound like ocean waves as you breathe.

Cooling Breath - seat yourself again. Roll your tongue into a tube (if you're a non-tongue roller, then simply pucker your lips). Then, stick out your tongue from between your lips and inhale through the tube formed by your tongue or mouth. It should be like pulling air in through a straw and filling your lungs with that air. Exhale through the nose with your mouth closed. Repeat multiple times (up to 26, although 5 or 10 can also work if you're pressed for time.)

Humming Bee Breath - Get seated again, close your eyes, and plug your ears with your fingers. Inhale, then exhale, making a humming buzz sound like a bee as you exhale. Make sure to keep your lips sealed the entire time and exhale for longer than you inhaled. Keep doing it anywhere from 5 to 15 times.

Integrating Breathing Into Poses

When you carry out your yoga, you carry out regular breathing rather than a dedicated breathing exercise. You should breathe diaphragmatic-ally before you start posing, then carry out the breathing during poses, inhaling when your chest opens up and inhaling when you compress it. Holding poses for about three calm breaths is also a good way to time yourself. Breathe deeply, and then, at the end of your exercise, use one of the breathing techniques while meditating as well.

Warming Up and Cooling Down

Traditional warmups are stretches that are done to prepare the body for physical exertion and some other manner of activity. It is essentially a mini practice or exercise before the actual activity that stretches and warms the body and muscles in preparation for the sorts of dynamic movements and actions it will be called to do.

A cool down is a purposeful transition that allows the body to come down from the highs of more intense physical activity to typical regular levels. Cooling down gives the body a gradual slowdown rather than an abrupt stop. It allows the heart rate to slow down and allows some pressure and tension relief from the muscles and joints. A cool-down is important to prevent injury and to stabilise post-workout blood flow.

Warm Up

For chair yoga, the process of warming up is just as important. To stay on brand, the warmups are altered a little from regular warmups to suit the chair that is so integral to the work we will be doing here.

The sweet spot for warming up (time-wise) is about five to 10 minutes of preliminary work to get the muscles warmed up and the stiffness out. This ensures some flexibility and joint mobility. The key to a good warmup is to start gently, making precise movements to increase circulation and movement.

Some basic stretches are all you need to do, really, while keeping a focus on breathing as well.

Reach Your Arms as Far Forward as you can (inhaling), keeping a 90-degree angle to the abdomen. Spread your arms out to your sides as wide open as you can (inhaling), then bring your arms together again (exhaling). Repeat five times for each side.

Stretch the Neck - Rock your head side to side and back and forth. Set aside that will be for inhaling, then a side that will be for exhaling. To do additional stretching, place your hands on the sides of your chair and repeat the process slowly and deliberately. (An alternate exercise is to turn the head to face the left and right directions, turning as far as is comfortable.) Repeat for 15 seconds.

Stretch the Sides - Reach one arm at a time up over your head toward the ceiling and then lean in the direction opposite where your arm is (Inhaling). Keep the arm raised and stretched when leaning. Keep the hips firmly placed on the seat. Then bring the arm down and bring your body out of the lean and back to the vertical position (exhaling. Repeat with each arm five times).

Roll the Shoulders - When rolling them up and backward, be sure to inhale. Then exhale as you bring them down and forward. Repeat the stretch 10 times.

Then, reverse the direction. Inhaling when the chest expands and exhaling when it contracts

Spine Stretches - Spread your legs wide and straighten your back with your palms resting on your lower thigh. Then lean forward, with the middle of your chest angled toward one of your knees (inhaling), then straighten again (exhaling). Lean forward again, center of the chest toward the other knee, and repeat. (to alternate, you can lean forward toward one knee, then complete a revolution where you lean toward the other knees in a single motion and then straighten again.) Be sure not to use your arms for support or put pressure on them; use your back muscles to support you. Repeat 10 times

Use the Seated Cat/Cow – as discussed already

Stretch Ankles - Center one of your feet and then stretch it out in front of you while keeping the other leg still. Start performing gentle ankle rolls on that foot. Pointing the toes forward and then up to the ceiling, making circles with your feet only, keeping the legs still. Make sure to wiggle the ankle back and forth while breathing rhythmically. Repeat for 10-15 seconds.

Seated Twists - Bring your arms forward again. While keeping vertical, reach out to one side, twisting the abdominal area (inhaling), then after holding for a little, come back to the normal position (exhaling). Afterwards, reach out in the other direction and come back to the normal position. Hold for five breaths on each side, then repeat these three to five times.

Leg Lifts - if you can lift your foot in the air and then put it down, lift the other foot and do the same, perform 10 repetitions for each leg. If you cannot lift your legs, then gently yet firmly slap the thighs to maximize circulation.

Cool Down

A good five to ten minutes should usually be enough to cool down as well. There are a few cool-down stretches that you can employ.

Seated Forward Fold - as already discussed.

Seated Butterfly - bring your legs together and push your knees apart. If you have any props to lift your legs, you can do that. (you want to come as close to sitting cross-legged as you can) then hold that pose. At intervals, apply a little bit of force to stretch the hips and the back. Hold the pose and breathe through it for 15 seconds.

Doing Some Light Power Walking is a Good Option - Take a walk, move briskly, make sure to swing your arms a little bit, and keep your back straight as you do it.

Meditation - this is controlled and focused breathing in a comfortable position.

You have learned the fundamentals of yoga; in the next chapter, you will learn a full yoga routine that contains some additional poses.

CHAPTER 5

BEGINNER WORKOUT: 20-MINUTE FULL BODY PROGRAM

With chair yoga, you can enhance your day and health with only a 20-minute routine right in the comfort of your home. The important action here is to prioritise consistency. Making sure you work out on a regular schedule is crucial to realising lasting results from these exercises.

WARM-UP ROUTINE

Having started with chair yoga fundamentals in the previous chapter, you are familiar with most, if not all, of these warm-up movements. In this beginner 20-minute workout, these movements will make up the entire warm-up sequence. Be sure to take this quick sequence seriously, as it gets your body prepared for the exercises and poses that are about to commence. Remember to prioritize breathing in every step throughout this workout and repeat it for a few days; once you feel it isn't pushing you, then move into a slightly more advanced routine.

Neck Stretches - Rock your head side to side and back and forth.

Set one side that will be for inhaling, then the opposite side that will be for exhaling. Hold each side for five-10 breaths.

To do additional stretching, place your hands on the sides of your chair and repeat the process slowly and deliberately. (An alternate exercise is to turn the head to face the left and right directions, turning as far as is comfortable.)

Shoulder Rolls - When rolling them up and backward, be sure to inhale.

Then exhale as you bring them down and forward.

Repeat the stretch a few times. Then, reverse the direction. Inhaling when the chest expands and exhaling when it contracts, perform five-10 rolls in each direction (forward and backward)

Seated Cat/Cow - Sit upright in your chair with your back straight.

Then, place your palms on your legs. You want to let your midsection lean back, pushing the hips and curving the back into a bit of a hunch.

Try to keep your head and shoulders in their initial position (just lowered) while the midsection curls backward, and you push your chest inward (inhaling).

Then come forward and, push your chest out, and tilt your head up, arching the back inward toward the thighs and knees (exhaling).

When you reach the maximum comfortable stretch on each inward/outward stretch, hold the pose for a little while, then release and slowly engage the other position.

The recommended duration for each pose/movement is listed below. Note that should you have a specific knot/stiffness in a particular area that the warm-up targets, you can go ahead and increase the number of repetitions for that muscle group to stretch out and alleviate the stiffness if possible.

Neck Stretches: Hold each side for 5-10 breaths

Shoulder Rolls: 5-10 rolls in each direction

Seated Cat/Cow: 5-10 repetitions

MAIN WORKOUT

Seated Eagle Arms - While seated vertically, fully stretch your arms out in front of you. Then, cross your right hand under and toward the left side of the left arm while still keeping them stretched out in front of you.

The next step is to bend your elbows in both arms to form something close to 90 degrees with angles pointing upwards.

After that, wrap both arms together and, applying most of the force with your right hand, lift your elbows up and simultaneously attempt to drop your shoulders.

You should feel some tension and pressure in your arms, shoulders, and upper back.

Hold for 5 -10 breaths, then repeat on the other side, simply opposing the order, having your left arm under the right.

Seated, Mountain Pose - Sit on a chair with your back straight and your feet firmly planted on the floor - shoulder width apart, rest your palms flat on your thighs.

Then, take a deep breath, extending your spine while simultaneously pushing your feet onto the floor (inhaling).

Then, as you start to exhale, draw your stomach in and allow your shoulders to slump a little. As you progress, include troubling the head to the left or right direction as you inhale to give the back muscles more of a stretch.

You can then repeat this exercise three to five times while being sure not to overextend yourself.

You should feel the back, core, and thigh muscles engaged in this use case.

Seated Side Bend - Reach one arm at a time up over your head toward the ceiling and then lean in the direction opposite where your arm is (Inhaling).

Keep the arm raised and stretched when leaning. Keep the hips firmly placed on the seat.

Then, bring the arm down and bring your body out of the lean and back to the vertical position (exhaling) Repeat with each arm in alternate turns about five times.

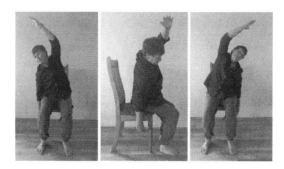

Seated Twist - for this pose, you will either want a chair without a backrest or, if it's removable, remove it; if you cannot do either, then move forward so you are sitting closer to the edge of your seat.

Again, centre yourself on the chair and breathe in deep. Raise your arms to about chest height and bend your elbows such that your palms are close to your chest.

You should then turn your upper body - chest, arms, head, etc to one side, keeping your hips firmly planted on the chair.

Hold for a few breaths, then slowly turn back toward the starting position. Then, repeat in the other direction. Carry out three to five twists on each side.

This exercise stretches the back muscles, the spine, the shoulders, and even the hips and glutes with the crossed leg variation.

If you want to raise the challenge of this exercise before starting, take one leg and cross it over the other. So, one thigh rests atop the other.

Then, perform the exercise, making sure that your hips remain on the seat. The leg that is lifted and crossed is pointing in the opposite direction to the direction you are turning to face.

For example, when turning to the left, you cross your left leg over your right. You can step it up even further by stretching out your arms and reaching out in the direction you are turning.

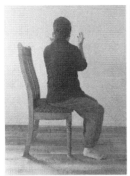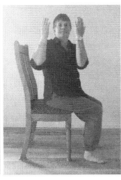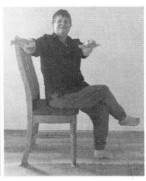

Seated Forward Bend - To maximise this pose, start yourself off in the already explained seated mountain pose.

Back straight, head elevated, feet pushing into the ground. Inhaling into the seated mountain, you then breathe out as you lean forward over your thighs.

In this pose, keep the arms at your sides if you can (keep them on your knees and then lower them to your shins if you need them to support you.)

Bend as far forward as you can without pain and hold that position for a few seconds, breathing deeply before coming back to the normal position in the upright seated mountain. Repeat three to five times.

Seated Forward Fold - Seat yourself upright in the chair and spread your legs about shoulder width apart, if not a little further, and inhale.

Then, you want to place the hands on the knees (initially), and as you start to exhale, you should bend forward from the hips, leaning your chest toward your knees.

As you lean, move your hands from your knees lower onto your shins and, if you can, keep going until they reach the floor. Without overexerting yourself, what you want to achieve is to be able to fold far enough ahead that your chest and midsection are essentially flat against your thighs and your hands are firmly on the floor.

Take care not to bend too far forward, as your head should remain on the same level as your knees in the pose's maximum stretch.

Going any further is an advanced technique with different instructions. Repeat three to five times.

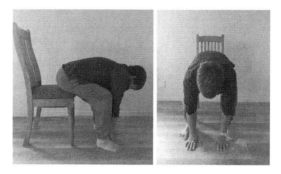

Seated Figure 4 Stretch - Center yourself on the chair with your feet touching the ground.

Then, lift one foot off the ground and place it over the knee to create a figure four with your legs. Keeping your back straight and your hips on the seat, lean forward over your thighs.

Do not arch your back as you lean; remain straight and bend from the hips. You should feel some pressure in the muscles around your hips and lower back, as well as the back of the thigh on the raised leg.

After holding for 20-30 seconds, rise and switch legs, doing the exact same stretch for the same period. Be sure to maintain proper posture and never bounce up and down during the exercise, as it can harm you.

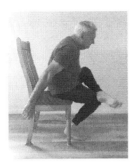 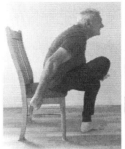 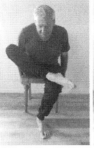 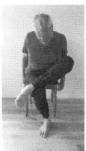

Wrist Stretches - Sit upright and extend one arm out in front of you. With your arm held out in front of you, start to slowly bend your wrist, pointing your hand towards the floor; as that hand is in that position, take your other hand and gently turn the wrist even further down until you feel some pressure in your forearms.

Hold in this position for 20 -30 seconds, and then release and work on the other wrist. Repeat five times.

Once you have done that, repeat the process of extending your arms and stretching the wrists, but point your hands upwards to the wall in front of you and use the other hand to pull your hand backward until you feel pressure.

For additional stretching, you can also carry out full wrist rolls, where you rotate your hands in 360-degree circles using your wrists. This should be done slowly and deliberately, and it is completely normal to hear a crack or two while doing this.

Another exercise that can accompany this is balling the hands into fists and then un-balling the fists and stretching the fingers. Repeat this process a few times.

Seated Tree Pose - There are multiple variations of the seated tree pose, but a simple one is to sit upright in your chair.

Then, raise one foot and place it over your knee. Then, bring your arms together into a prayer pose at chest height. You want to inhale while doing this, then exhale as you raise your arms up and above your head. Hold for three to five deep breaths.

If you can, you want the arch that is created by your raised arms to be directly overhead, with your arms fully stretched. Hold there for some time, and then lower them to your chest again.

You can then switch which leg is raised and crossing the other and cycle through a few repetitions.

If that is challenging, you can initially execute the pose without lifting the leg and resting it over your knee. Hold for three to five deep breaths.

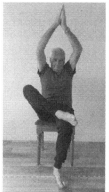 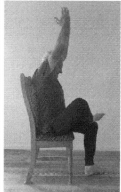 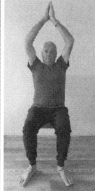 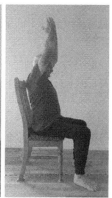

Knee to Chest - Sit upright in the chair with your feet flat on the floor. Place your hands underneath one thigh.

Using the force of your arms, lift your thigh toward your chest, only going as far as you comfortably can while keeping your hips on the chair.

Be sure to keep your head and your chest straight while practising this pose. Hold this pose for a few seconds, and then lower your leg slowly and lift the other toward your chest again.

If you can lift the leg toward your chest without solely relying on your hands, then you can do so. Repeat 5 - 10 times.

Do not rest the sole on the edge of the seat, as that invalidates the stretch.

Ankle Stretches - Center one of your feet, lift it and stretch it out in front of you. Then, start performing gentle ankle rolls on that foot.

Pointing the toes forward and then up to the ceiling, making circles with your feet only, keeping the legs still. Make sure to wiggle the ankle back and forth while breathing rhythmically. Repeat for 15 seconds.

If you wish to do it with more control, you can raise one leg and cross over the other knee and then use your hands to manually stretch the ankle by manipulating the foot, pointing the toes away from you, pulling them towards you, etc.

Seated Calf Raise - For the exercise, you want to sit forward on your chair as much as you can while still being reasonably comfortable.

Then you want to hold onto the sides of your chairs, and using the muscles in the foot, you want to raise your heels off the ground until you are only being supported by your toes.

Your knees should be elevated above your hips and off the chair completely. Do this as far as you can, aiming at supporting your legs on your tippy toes.

Then hold for a few seconds and then return to normal; in that process, rock back onto the soles of your feet, raise your front foot, and try to point your toes toward the ceiling.

After a few seconds, return your feet to a flat stance and repeat the process. Throughout both exercises, you should feel tension in your calves.

Seated Hamstring Stretch - Again, move toward the front edge of your chair. Then, you want to stretch one leg out in front of you as much as you can while keeping your back straight and your head upright.

Then, you want to slowly lean forward, bending at the hips again as you move your chest toward your knees.

Keep doing this until you feel pressure at the back of your thigh, and then hold around that area for 15 seconds.

You will notice your ability to comfortably bend further forward increasing as time goes on.

Upper Back Stretch - Sit upright in your chair. You want to reach your arms forward and clasp them together.

While keeping a straight back, you want to reach as far forward as you can with those outstretched hands and also lean forward with your head and shoulders.

For further stretching, you can adopt a diving pose with your hands, where you place one hand atop the other like you would before diving into some water.

Hold the outstretched pose for 15 seconds and then release and slowly return to your regular position.

Chest Expansion - in your regular seated position, grip the back corner area of your chair with your arms. Breathe in and then exhale.

After exhaling, push your chest outwards and upward (inhaling), curving the back a little bit and rolling the shoulders back as well.

Push as far forward as you comfortably can, feeling some pressure in the chest muscles. Hold for three to five breaths and then return to normal position. Repeat three to five times.

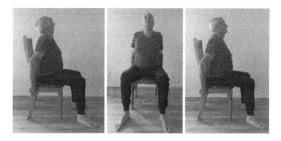

Cool Down Routine

Seated Meditation - Keep your breathing in check and practice a breathing exercise while you clear your mind and focus on mental and physical harmony; refer to Chapter 4 to learn some breathing techniques that will help you with this meditation.

Final Relaxation: Body Scan - As you meditate or take a short walk to cool down, make sure to conduct an overall body scan and wellness check. Is there any new muscle or joint soreness from the exercise? If not, do any aches and pains you previously had feel any better?

Conduct this audit on your body every time before and after an exercise. If you develop new pain, it might be a sign you are doing a pose wrong or are not aligned, or it might signify an undiagnosed issue in that region.

If you had pain before exercising, take it easy when engaging in exercises that include that joint or muscle group.

The duration of the entire cool-down phase is about three to five minutes, sometimes 10.

You have now learned a beginner full-body yoga workout program. Next, we will look into another yoga routine that contains some different poses.

Chapter 6

Beginner Workout: 30-Minute Full Body Program

Half an hour a day equals a lifetime of benefits! It's a pretty sensational Return On Investment if you ask me, and I believe that you agree as well.

WARMUP

The focus during the warmup should remain on breathing exercises and extended stretches. If you are very comfortable, then you can extend the duration and difficulty of the exercises or pose. When transitioning between exercises, make sure to return to the normal base upright seating in the chair before you engage in a new exercise or stretch.

Neck Stretches - Gently tilt your head side to side and forward/back to loosen the neck.

Hold each stretch for five breaths.

Shoulder Rolls - Seated upright, lift your shoulders towards your ears.

Then, roll your shoulders backward and downwards toward the natural resting state. Make sure to feel some pressure in your neck and upper back. Repeat 5 times.

Seated Cat/Cow - Place your palms on your legs. You want to let your midsection lean back, pushing the hips and curving the back into a bit of a hunch.

Try to keep your head and shoulders in their initial position (just lowered) while the midsection curls backward, and you push your chest inward (inhaling).

Then, come forward, push your chest out, and tilt your head up, arching the back inward toward the thighs and knees (exhaling).

Ankle Circles - While seated, lift one foot and the floor and draw a circle with your foot, rotating it at the ankle joint.

Be sure that the rest of your leg does not move and that only the foot moves.

Slowly draw the circle with each foot and ankle five times clockwise and five times counter-clockwise, then switch foot.

Wrist Circles - full wrist rolls where you rotate your hands in 360 circles using your wrists.

This should be done slowly and deliberately, and it is completely normal to hear a crack or two while doing this.

Extend arms out and circle wrists five times clockwise and five times counter-clockwise.

Overhead Reach - Inhale deeply, then raise your arms and reach up toward the ceiling as far as you comfortably can.

You should feel some pull in your back and your arms.

Hold for 5 -10 seconds, and then lower your arms again. Repeat five times.

Seated Twist - For this pose, you will either want a chair without a backrest or, if it's removable, remove it; if you cannot do either, then move forward so you are sitting closer to the edge of your seat.

Again, centre yourself on the chair and breathe in deeply. Raise your arms to about chest height and bend your elbows such that your palms are close to your chest.

You should then turn your upper body - chest, arms, head, etc to one side, keeping your hips firmly planted on the chair. Hold for five breaths, then slowly turn back toward the starting position.

Then, repeat in the other direction for five turns.

This exercise stretches the back muscles, the spine, the shoulders, and even the hips and glutes with the crossed leg variation. If you cannot raise your arms, then place one on your knees and the other behind you, then turn to the side.

Main Workout

Mountain Pose - Sit on a chair with your back straight and your feet firmly planted on the floor - shoulder width apart, rest your palms flat on your thighs.

Then, take a deep breath, extending your spine while simultaneously pushing your feet onto the floor (inhaling).

Then, as you start to exhale, draw your stomach in and allow your shoulders to slump a little

As you progress, include turning the head to the left or right direction as you inhale to give the back muscles more of a stretch. Hold for 5 - 10 seconds.

Warrior I - While in a seated mountain pose (refer to chapter five), turn your body to the left side so that your backrest is now on your left.

Next, take your right leg and stick it out behind you, as far back as it can go.

Then, keep your left leg on the chair with a 90-degree bend in the knee, raise your arms above your head, and clasp your palms together.

If you are struggling with sticking out the right(back) leg behind, you can stick it out to the side instead, and when you build up, move it further back.

Hold the pose for five breaths. Then, switch sides.

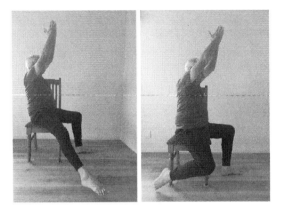

Forward Fold - Seat yourself upright in the chair, spread your legs about shoulder width apart, if not a little further, and inhale.

Then, you want to place the hands on the knees (initially), and as you start to exhale, you should bend forward from the hips, leaning your chest toward your knees.

As you lean, move your hands from your knees lower onto your shins and, if you can, reach the floor. Without overexerting yourself, what you want to achieve is to be able to fold far enough ahead that your chest and midsection are flat against your knees.

Hold for five breaths.

Half Forward Fold -Similar to a forward fold, but you initially raise your arms above your head.

Then, instead of bending to the point where you almost lie flat against your thighs, bend to about halfway (45 degrees).

Using your hips as a hinge point and with your arms still raised, hold the pose for five breaths.

Repeat two-three times.

Extended Leg Stretch - Sitting upright, lift one of your legs up and hold it out straight in front of you.

You should feel some pressure in your thigh as you do it. Then, while holding that leg out straight, reach out with one (or both) arm(s) for your toes.

Reach as far forward as you can with the goal being touching your toes, then hold for five breaths, after which switch sides.

Take care not to overdo it, as it can cause back and hamstring problems if you do.

Warrior II - Repeat the same procedure as Warrior I, where you stick one leg to the side and then raise your arms.

The difference is that in this pose, you spread your arms out at your sides rather than over your head, and you do not turn to the side but do this one straight on.

With arms spread, back straight, and palms down,

Hold for five breaths, then switch sides.

Eagle Arms - While seated vertically, fully stretch your arms forward in front of you.

Then, cross your right hand under and toward the left side of the left arm while still stretched out in front of you.

The next step is to bend your elbows in both arms to form something close to 90-degree angles pointing upwards.

After that, wrap both arms together and, applying most of the force with your right hand, lift your elbows up and simultaneously attempt to drop your shoulders.

Hold for five breaths. Switch sides.

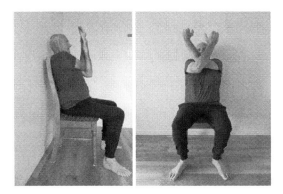

Seated Twist - Procedure as already detailed in chapter four. Place your right hand on your left knee and your left hand behind you. Twist the torso to the left. Hold for five breaths. Switch sides.

Seated Cat/Cow - Procedure as already described in chapter four. Inhale, arch back and look up. Exhale, round back, and look down, then repeat five times.

Bridge Pose - Starting with a seated mountain pose, hold the sides of the chair you are sitting on and make sure your feet are firmly placed flat on the ground.

Then, using your arms to support you, lift your hips up off the chair and slowly thrust forward.

Push far out to create a bridge pose, where from your legs up to your head, there should be a smooth, almost convex arch.

Hold for five breaths, then repeat twice.

In this pose, only go as far out as you can; if you have back issues or knee issues that make this a problem, then do not engage in it.

Boat Pose - In this pose, you are again on a seated mountain (as described in chapter five). You want to grip the sides of your chair with your hands to start.

Raise both knees up above the seat into an inclined position and lean back in your chair. Keep your legs suspended in the air without additional support and hold.

For those who feel able to, you can then straighten your legs to remove the bend in your knees and make the legs completely straight as well as not resting on the chair backrest when you lean back (which is challenging and only recommended if you are sure you can do it).

Hold for 10 seconds. Repeat five times.

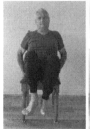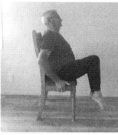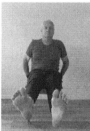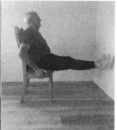

Tree Pose - sit upright in your chair. Then again, raise one foot and place it over your knee. Then, bring your arms together into a prayer pose at chest height.

You want to inhale while doing this, then exhale as you raise your arms up and above your head. If you can, you want the arch that was created to be directly overhead, with your arms straight.

Hold there for some time, and then lower them down to your chest again. You can then switch the leg that is raised, cross the other, and cycle through a few repetitions.

If that is challenging, you can initially execute the pose without lifting the leg and resting it over your knee.

Hold for 10 seconds. Switch sides.

Extended Side Stretch - Reach one arm at a time up over your head toward the ceiling and then lean in the direction opposite where your arm is (Inhaling).

Keep the arm raised and stretched when leaning. Keep the hips firmly placed on the seat.

Then, bring the arm down and bring your body out of the lean and back to the vertical position. Hold for 5 breaths.

Seated Spinal Twist - Like the seated bend from chapter five, but with a minor alternation. Cross right knee over left. Place your left hand behind you and your right hand on your right knee. Twist to the right. Hold for five breaths. Switch sides.

Seated Crescent Moon - Like the extended side stretch from chapter five but with a variation.

Inhale, extend arms out to sides, palms up.

Exhale, reach your right hand overhead and left hand back behind you.

Hold for five breaths. Switch sides.

Shoulder Shrugs - Lift shoulders up toward ears, hold for a breath, then release and allow them to come down.

Inhale when the arms are lowered, exhale when they are raised, and contract the chest. Repeat five times.

Neck Stretches - Rock your head from side to side and back and forth.

Set one side that will be for inhaling, then the opposite side that will be for exhaling.

To do additional stretching, place your hands on the sides of your chair and repeat the process slowly and deliberately. (An alternate exercise is to turn the head to face the left and right directions, turning as far as is comfortable.)

Hold each stretch for five breaths.

Seated Yogic Breathing - Sit tall with eyes closed. Do diaphragmatic breathing as described in chapter five.

Cool Down

Ankle Circles - Procedure as already detailed. Lift your feet off the floor and circle your ankles five times clockwise and five times counterclockwise.

Wrist Circles - Procedure as already detailed above. Extend your arms out and circle your wrists five times clockwise and five times counterclockwise.

Seated Twist - centre yourself on the chair and breathe in deeply. Raise your arms to about chest height and bend your elbows such that your palms are close to your chest. You should then turn your upper body - chest, arms, head, etc. to one side, keeping your hips firmly planted on the chair. Hold for a few breaths, then slowly turn back toward the starting position. Hold for five breaths. Repeat on the other side.

Seated Cat/Cow - As described above. Inhale, arch back and look up. Exhale, round back, and look down. Repeat five times.

Seated Meditation - Sit tall with eyes closed. Take five deep breaths.

You have now learned a second full beginner yoga routine; we will look to step it up and increase the challenge and length of the routines.

MAKE A DIFFERENCE WITH YOUR REVIEW

UNLOCK THE POWER OF GENEROSITY

"Yoga is when every cell in the body sings the song of the soul." — *B.K.S IYENGAR*

Hey there!

A few years ago, in my mid-sixties, I felt the toll of aging. The persistent aches and non-physical exhaustion were daily companions. Despite a good life and regular walks, I knew things could be better. Surprisingly, just half an hour of exercise per week changed my life for the better......

Now, let's talk about you. Would you help someone you've never met, even if you never got credit for it?

Who is this person you ask? They are like you. Or, at least, like you used to be. Less experienced, wanting to make a difference, and needing help, but not sure where to look.

Our mission is to make "Chair Yoga for Seniors" accessible to everyone. Everything I do stems from that mission. And, the only way for me to accomplish that mission is by reaching... well...everyone.

This is where you come in. Most people do judge a book by its cover (and its reviews). So here's my ask on behalf of a struggling senior you've never met:

Please help that senior by leaving this book a review.

Your gift costs no money and less than 60 seconds to make, but can change a fellow senior's life forever. Your review could help...

One more small business provides for their community. One more entrepreneur supports their family. One more employee gets meaningful work. One more client transformed their life.

One more dream come true.

To get that 'feel good' feeling and help this person for real, all you have to do is...and it takes less than 60 seconds... leave a review.

If you feel good about helping a faceless senior, you are my kind of person. Welcome to the club. You're one of us.

I'm that much more excited to help you find relief, balance, and independence than you can possibly imagine. You'll love the empowering poses I'm about to share in the coming chapters.

Thank you from the bottom of my heart. Now, back to our regularly scheduled programming.

Your biggest fan, Laurel Harris

Scan the QR code to leave your review!

Chapter 7

Intermediate Workout: 20-30 Minutes Full Body Program

Are you ready to level up? Because if you've gone this far, your body and mind are definitely ready. It is important to understand that some of the intermediate exercises are beginner exercises that are held for a longer period or have some additional elements, such as weights or resistance bands, added on to give additional complexity.

INTERMEDIATE WARMUP

Dynamic Stretches are an important aspect of the process that you will go through; these are types of stretches that revolve around the movement of the muscle to bring about the stretching rather than simply holding a pose (static stretching).

Seated Cat/cow Stretches - Place your palms on your legs. You want to let your midsection lean back, pushing the hips and curving the back into a bit of a hunch.

Try to keep your head and shoulders in their initial position (just lowered) while the midsection curls backward, and you push your chest inward (inhaling).

Then come forward and, push your chest out, and tilt your head up, arching the back inward toward the thighs and knees (exhaling).

Repeat five times.

Neck Stretches - Rock your head side to side and back and forth.

Set one side that will be for inhaling, then the opposite side that will be for exhaling.

To do additional stretching, place your hands on the sides of your chair and repeat the process slowly and deliberately. (An alternate exercise is to turn the head to face the left and right directions, turning as far as is comfortable.)

Hold each stretch for five breaths.

Shoulder Rolls - Sit upright, lift your shoulders towards your ears, and then hold for a little while.

Then, roll your shoulders backward and downwards toward the natural resting state.

Make sure to feel some pressure in your neck and upper back.

Repeat five times.

Seated Twists - Center yourself on the chair and breathe in deep. Raise your arms to about chest height and bend your elbows such that your palms are close to your chest and your elbows are sticking out in either direction (like chicken wings).

You should then turn your upper body - chest, arms, head, etc to one side, keeping your hips firmly planted on the chair.

Hold for a few breaths, then slowly turn back toward the starting position. Then, repeat in the other direction for a few turns.

This exercise stretches the back muscles, the spine, the shoulders, and even the hips and glutes with the crossed leg variation.

If you cannot raise your arms, then place one on your knees and the other behind you, then turn to the side.

Hold for thirty seconds, and then repeat three times.

Ankle Circles - While seated, lift one foot and the floor and draw a circle with your foot, rotating it at the ankle joint.

Be sure that the rest of your leg does not move and that only the foot moves. Slowly draw the circle with each foot and ankle five times clockwise and five times counterclockwise, then switch feet.

CORE WORKOUT

Intermediate-Level Warrior II - seated mountain pose from chapter four.

Next up, take your right leg and stick it out behind you, as far back as it can go. Keep your left leg on the chair with a 90-degree bend in the knee.

Spread your arms out at your sides and raise them to the point where they are in line with your chest, creating what looks like extended wings at full stretch.

Keep your torso aligned vertically, being sure not to bend it in either direction.

With arms spread, back straight, and palms down, hold for 30 seconds, then switch sides.

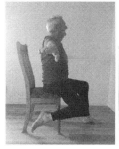
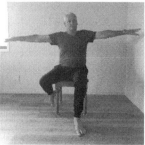

Extended Side Angle - Spread your legs to the point where they are placed on either side of the chair you are sitting on.

Then, stretch out one leg as far as possible, feeling some tension in your hamstrings, while the foot on the other leg is flat on the floor and maintains a 90-degree bend in the knee joint.

Then, reach one arm at a time up over your head toward the ceiling and then lean toward your 90-degree knee. Keep the arm raised and stretched when leaning. Keep the hips firmly placed on the seat.

Then, bring the arm down and bring your body out of the lean and back to the vertical position.

Ideally, you should have a straight-ish line formed by the outside of your extended leg, to your torso, and up to the extended arm.

Hold for 30 seconds on each side.

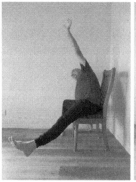
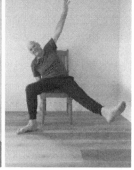

Intermediate Level Chair Pigeon - In the seated mountain pose, lift one leg and cross it over the other so one leg's ankle rests over the knee of the other.

Hinging at the hips, lean forward with the back still straight so your torso and chest approach your knees. You are essentially forward folding.

Keep the hips flat on the chair and then switch to the other leg being crossed over and repeat.

Hold the pose for 30 seconds, with each leg crossing over the other.

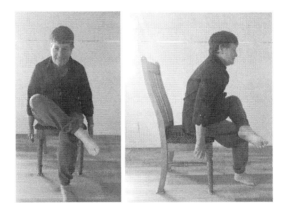

Intermediate Level Seated Forward Bend - Seat yourself upright in the chair and spread your legs about shoulder width apart, if not a little further, and inhale.

Then, you want to place the hands on the knees (initially), and as you start to exhale, you should bend forward from the hips, leaning your chest toward your knees (hinge your body at the hips and fold over).

As you lean forward, move your hands from your knees lower onto your shins and, if you can, all the way until you reach the floor.

Without overexerting yourself, what you want to achieve is to be able to fold far enough ahead that your chest and midsection are flat against your knees.

Hold for 30 seconds.

Intermediate Level Seated Twist - for this pose, you will either want a chair without a backrest or, if it's removable, remove it; if you cannot do either, then move forward so you are sitting closer to the edge of your seat.

Again, centre yourself on the chair and breathe in deeply. Raise your arms to about chest height and bend your elbows such that your palms are close to your chest.

You should then turn your upper body - chest, arms, head, etc to one side, keeping your hips firmly planted on the chair. Then, slowly turn back toward the starting position.

Then, repeat in the other direction.

This exercise stretches the back muscles, the spine, the shoulders, and even the hips and glutes with the crossed leg variation.

Hold each side for 30 seconds, then switch to the other side.

Intermediate-Level Eagle Arms - While seated vertically, fully stretch your arms forward in front of you.

Then, cross your right hand under and toward the left side of the left arm while still remaining stretched out in front of you.

The next step is to bend your elbows and pull the lower arm section in both hands toward you to form something close to 90-degree angles pointing upwards.

After that, wrap both arms together and, applying most of the force with your right hand, lift your elbows up and simultaneously attempt to drop your shoulders.

Hold for 30 seconds. Then, switch sides.

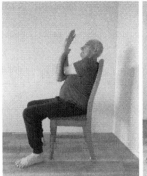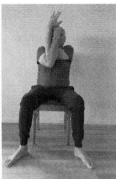

Seated Rows - You will need some equipment for this one; slowly grab some full half or one-litre water bottles or some light weights.

Sit upright with your back straight. Grab the weights and have them in your arms. Relax the shoulders and arms, keeping them flat at your sides with the weights in them.

Brace your core, lift the arms, and extend them directly out in front of you to just below chest height.

Using your core and keeping your arms raised, draw the elbows back toward you in a rowing motion. Right until they are just past your torso, then hold. Be sure to keep a straight back; do not lean backward.

Slowly extend the arms back out again without leaning forward. Be sure, to do both pulling and pushing out with your back muscles and not your arms.

Carry out 10 slow and deliberate repetitions, monitoring your breathing as you go about it.

Overhead Press - Again, hold your weights in your hands.

Start with a straight back, arms loose and by your sides, feet flat on the ground. Keep your glutes, back, and neck all in line.

Nice, and slowly lift your weights from the default position to your shoulder level, being sure to implement a reverse (pronated) grip on the weights (palms facing upward). Keep the dumbbells at shoulder width or a little further away without exertion. This is your resting position.

Press (push) the dumbbells upwards and overhead to the full extension of your arms. The arms should ideally be fully extended vertically above your head in a straight manner. Also, do not arch your lower back at any point.

Lower the dumbbells in a controlled fashion, bending your elbows until they return to the rest position. Repeat for ten deliberate repetitions.

Triceps Kickbacks - Again, grab some weights and start in a seated position with back straight arms down at your sides.

Hinge yourself at the hips and lean forward over the knees. Keep your arms in line with your torso, and as you bend, keep the arms straight so that they are at the same angle as your torso.

Then, lift the weights toward your chest a little so that your elbows form a ninety-degree angle, keeping your bicep upper arm in line with the torso still.

Extend your arms backward using your forearm, straightening your arms in the process. Once your arms are fully extended, hold for 5 seconds. You should feel some pressure in your triceps doing this.

Return to the start position slowly, bending the elbows and pulling the weights towards your chest.

Repeat for ten deliberate repetitions.

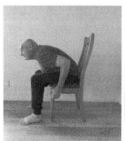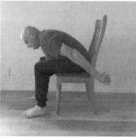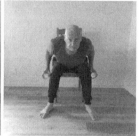

Intermediate level Seated Marching - In the default seated mountain pose, without weights and arms down at the sides.

Keep your hips flat in the chair and lift one knee above the floor toward the ceiling. Raise it to a comfortable level about 45 degrees from the horizontal.

Then, lower the knee and switch to and raise the other.

Keep alternating between both knees in a sort of marching rhythm.

Repeat the slow and deliberate marching motion for 30 seconds.

Ankle Pumps - sit upright with your back straight and feet flat on the ground.

Place your palms on your knees, making sure they are in line with your hips, and create a 90-degree angle to the floor.

Lift your heels off the ground and into the air, supporting your legs only by the front section of your toes. Your knees should rise above your hips at this point.

Hold for a second and then release and return feet to their natural position.

Repeat the slow and deliberate pumping motion for 30 seconds.

Cooling Down

Seated Twist - Repeat as already instructed in the warmup section of this chapter, holding each side for 30 seconds.

Seated Forward Bend - start yourself off in the already explained seated mountain pose. Back straight, head elevated, feet pushing into the ground.

Inhaling into the seated mountain, you then breathe out as you lean forward over your thighs.

In this pose, keep your arms at your sides if you can (keep them on your knees and then lower them to your shins if you need them to support you.)

Bend as far forward as you can without pain and hold that position for five seconds, breathing deeply before coming back to the normal position in the upright seated mountain. Hold for 15 seconds.

Eagle Arms - While seated vertically, fully stretch your arms forward in front of you. Then, cross your right hand under and toward the left side of the left arm while still stretched out in front of you.

The next step is to bend your elbows in both arms to form something close to 90-degree angles pointing upwards.

After that, wrap both arms together and, applying most of the force with your right hand, lift your elbows up and simultaneously attempt to drop your shoulders.

Hold for five breaths. Switch sides.

"Hands in Prayer" - Bring your hands to the centre of your chest and close your eyes. Try to clear your mind and focus on your body. Hold for three minutes.

Seated Meditation - Sit comfortably, close your eyes, and focus on your breathing. Hold for one-three minutes.

With these exercises, you have now stepped up the intensity and raised the bar on what you are able to do and accomplish. You must keep working to ascend past this intermediate level, as it doesn't stop here; there's more to be done, and more you are capable of.

Chapter 8

Intermediate Workout: 30-40 Minutes Full Body Program

You've come this far; now go even further!

INTERMEDIATE WARM-UP

Seated Cat/Cow Stretch - Place your palms on your legs. You want to let your midsection lean back, pushing the hips and curving the back into a bit of a hunch.

Try to keep your head and shoulders in their initial position (just lowered) while the midsection curls backward, and you push your chest inward (inhaling).

Then come forward and, push your chest out and tilt your head up, arching the back inward toward the thighs and knees (exhaling). Repeat 5 times.

Neck Stretches - Rock your head side to side and back and forth. Set one side that will be for inhaling, then the opposite side that will be for exhaling.

To do additional stretching, place your hands on the sides of your chair and repeat the process slowly and deliberately.

An alternate exercise is to turn the head to face the left and right directions, turning as far as is comfortable.

Hold each stretch for five breaths.

Shoulder Rolls - Move the shoulders upwards and backward, then downwards and forwards to form a complete circle; repeat the process without stopping. When rolling them up and backward, be sure to inhale.

Then exhale as you bring them down and forward.

Repeat the stretch five times.

Then, reverse the direction. Inhale when the chest expands and exhale when it contracts.

Seated Spinal Twist - Like the seated bend but with a minor alternation. Cross right knee over left.

Place your left hand behind you and your right hand on your right knee. Twist to the right.

Hold for five breaths. Switch sides.

Seated Eagle Arms - Fully stretch your arms forward in front of you. Then, cross your right hand under and toward the left side of the left arm while still stretched out in front of you.

The next step is to bend your elbows in both arms to form something close to 90-degree angles pointing upwards.

After that, wrap both arms together and, applying most of the force with your right hand, lift your elbows up and simultaneously attempt to drop your shoulders.

Hold for five breaths. Switch sides.

Ankle Circles - While seated, lift one foot off the floor and draw a circle with your foot, rotating it at the ankle joint.

Be sure that the rest of your leg does not move and that only the foot moves.

Slowly draw the circle with each foot and ankle five times clockwise and five times counterclockwise, then switch feet.

Seated Mountain Pose - Sit on a chair with your back straight and your feet firmly planted on the floor - shoulder width apart, rest your palms flat on your thighs.

Then, take a deep breath, extending your spine while simultaneously pushing your feet onto the floor (inhaling). Then, as you start to exhale, draw your stomach in and allow your shoulders to slump a little.

As you progress, include turning the head to the left or right direction as you inhale to give the back muscles more of a stretch. Hold for 5 deep breaths.

CORE WORKOUT

Chair Cat/Cow - Carry out as already mentioned in the warm-up.

Extended Leg Stretch - Start in the basic seated mountain. You want your arms either in your lap or if you need extra stability, you can place them on the sides of the chair.

Lift one foot and stretch it out in front of you as far forward as you can. You want to then flex the foot, pointing the toes upward and, if possible, toward you a little. This movement should stretch your hamstring.

Hold the pose while you continue to stretch and flex the foot. Then, lower the foot and repeat the process with the other foot.

As a variation, you can make the pose easier by not lifting the foot, simply moving forward in your chair and extending it as far forward as you can, with the foot remaining on the floor but stretching the hamstring regardless.

Repeat the same flexing and pointing of the foot and toes, hold for 30 seconds on each side, and repeat two times on each side.

Chair Warrior I - While in a seated mountain pose, turn your body to the left side so that your backrest is now on your left.

After that, take your right leg and stick it out behind you, as far back as it can go.

Then, keep your left leg on the chair with a 90-degree bend in the knee, raise your arms above your head, and clasp your palms together.

If you are struggling with sticking out the right (back) leg behind you, you can stick it out to the side instead and then build up to moving it further back.

Hold the pose for five breaths. Then, switch sides.

Chair Warrior II - Repeat the same procedure as Warrior I, where you stick one leg behind you, then raise your arms.

The difference is that in this pose, you spread your arms out at your sides rather than over your head, and you do not turn to the side but do this one straight on.

With arms spread, back straight, and palms down, hold for five breaths, then switch sides.

Chair Triangle - Set yourself in the seated mountain position, arms down at your sides and your back straight.

Then, lift one arm and raise it above your head as high as you possibly can.

Move the other and place it on the side of the chair down by your side. Extend the arms as much as you can; you should feel some pressure on your side as you do this. It is intended to stretch the sides.

After holding for thirty seconds, alternate the hand position to ensure both sides get a stretch.

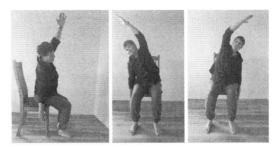

Chair Warrior III - Starting in the seated mountain position with your arms down by your sides.

Turn your whole body again to face either your left or right side. Make sure your knees are bent at 90 degrees, and your feet touch the ground. Extend one leg as far backward as you can.

Lift your arms from down by your sides and stretch them out in front of you as far forward as you can. You should feel some pressure in your hips and tension in your back if you are stretching enough.

Be sure to keep your back straight and keep your head in line with your body.

Hold for thirty seconds, then perform a 180-degree, half revolution on the chair, stretch out the other leg behind you and repeat the rest of the process.

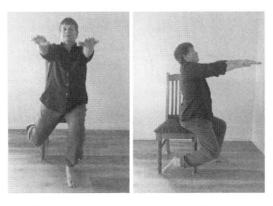

Chair Tree Pose - There are multiple variations of the seated tree pose, but a simple one is to sit upright in your chair.

Then again, raise one foot and place it over your knee. Then, bring your arms together into a prayer pose at chest height. You want to inhale while doing this, then exhale as you raise your arms up and above your head.

If you can, you want the arch that is created by your raised arms to be directly overhead, with your arms fully stretched. Hold there for 30 seconds, and then lower them to your chest again.

You can then switch the leg that is raised across the other and repeat five times on each side.

If that is challenging, you can initially execute the pose without lifting the leg and resting it over your knee.

Chair Dancer - Starting in the seated mountain position with your arms down by your sides. Turn your whole body again to face either your left or right side.

Make sure your knees are bent at 90 degrees, and your feet touch the ground. Extend one leg as far backward as you can.

Lift one arm (the arm that is opposite the leg you have stretched out behind you) from down by your side and stretch it out overhead.

Your body should resemble a dancer holding a pose as you do this. You should feel some pressure in your hips and tension in your back if you are stretching enough.

Be sure to keep your back straight and keep your head in line with your body.

Hold for thirty seconds, then turn on the chair and stretch out the other leg behind you, then repeat the rest of the process. Hold for 15 seconds on each side two times.

Seated Forward Bend - Seat yourself upright in the chair, spread your legs about shoulder width apart, if not a little further, and inhale.

Then, you want to place the hands on the knees (initially), and as you start to exhale, you should bend forward from the hips, leaning your chest toward your knees.

As you lean, move your hands from your knees lower onto your shins and, if you can, reach the floor.

Without overexerting yourself, what you want to achieve is to be able to fold far enough ahead that your chest and midsection are flat against your knees.

Hold for five breaths.

Seated Spinal Twist - Carry out as already mentioned in the warm-up. Hold for three to five breaths, then repeat three to five times.

Seated Eagle Arms - Carry out as already mentioned in the warm-up. Hold for three to five breaths, then repeat three to five times.

Chair Downward Facing Dog - Starting in the default seated mountain pose, with arms down by your sides, move forward to sit toward the edge of the chair.

Extend your legs out in front of you as far as you can. Make the entire leg straight while keeping only the heel in contact with the ground during this.

Then, using the hip joint as a hinge, fold forward slightly and reach your arms out as far forward as you can, or if possible, reach them out further above your head, keeping the reaching arms in line with your ears so that they are at the same angle as you are leaning forward.

Spread your shoulders a little bit, moving them away from your ears, and keep your eyes fixed on a specified spot on the ground in front of you or even inward toward your navel area.

Lean as far forward as you need to to bring your palms in line with your feet/toes so that it mimics how they would be in line were they both touch the ground in a standard downward-facing dog.

Hold for thirty seconds.

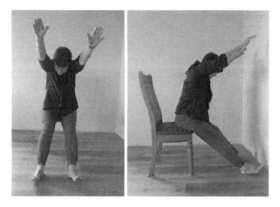

Chair Pigeon - In the seated mountain pose, lift one leg and cross it over the other so one leg's ankle rests over the knee of the other.

Hinging at the hips, lean forward with the back still straight so your torso and chest approach your knees.

You are essentially forward folding. Keep the hips flat on the chair and then switch to the other leg being crossed over and repeat.

Hold 30 seconds on each side.

Boat Pose - In this pose, you are again in a seated mountain. To start with, you want to grip the sides of your chair with your hands.

Raise both knees above the seat into an inclined position and lean back in your chair. Keep your legs suspended in the air without additional support and hold.

For those who are able, you can then straighten your legs to remove the bend in your knees and make the legs completely straight, as well as not resting on the chair backrest when you lean back (which is challenging and only recommended if you are sure you can do it).

Hold for 10 seconds. Repeat five times.

Bridge Pose - Start with a seated mountain pose; hold the sides of the chair you are sitting on, and make sure your feet are firmly placed flat on the ground.

Then, using your arms to support you, lift your hips up off the chair and slowly thrust forward.

Push far out to create a bridge pose, where from your legs up to your head, there should be a smooth, almost convex arch.

Hold for five breaths, then repeat twice.

In this pose, only go as far out as you can; if you have back issues or knee issues that make this a problem, then do not engage in it.

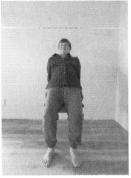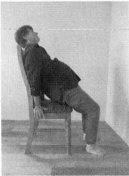

Seated Mountain Pose - Carry out as already mentioned in the warm-up. Hold for five breaths, then repeat three times.

Chair Sun Salutations - Ideally, it would work best if you had a window that faced wherever the sun was during your workout, but anywhere will do.

Sit towards the edge of the chair with your feet on the ground and knees at 90-degree angles. Keep your spine straight and bring your hands into a prayer position in front of your chest.

Then, raise the arms up as far as you can above your head.

Arms are in line with your ears and stretching until the elbows are straight. You can lean backward a little to push your chest out as you do so. Next, you bend forward slowly and reach your arms toward the ground.

The torso is fully flat against the thighs, and you should try to touch the ground in between and a little in front of your feet. After holding it, rise slowly toward your straightened pose again with your arms above your head.

Hold for 30 seconds.

An additional variation is that once you complete the exercise, take turns raising each knee toward the chest by placing your palms underneath each leg and pulling and lifting it toward your chest. Once you have done one turn of each leg, raise your arms into the prayer position and prepare to repeat the pose.

Seated Eagle Legs - The eagle's legs pose involves folding your legs in a pose similar to the eagle's arms as follows.

Start at the standard seated mountain pose, arms down by your sides.

Lift one leg and cross it over the other leg. Then, apply some pressure to the legs as they are crossed while holding the pose.

This should stretch the hips, thighs, and even the lower back a bit.

Hold for five to ten seconds and repeat three to five times.

Cool Down

Meditation

Find a comfortable seated position, close your eyes, and relax your body from head to toe. Focus on softening the muscles and calming the mind. Breathe slowly and deeply.

Scan the body for areas of tension. Consciously relax those areas on each exhale. Stay in this deep state of relaxation for up to 10 minutes.

This is the next evolution of your yoga workout. It is important not to stagnate but to keep improving slowly over time and develop more flexibility and endurance. There is no defined ceiling on the benefits that can be achieved through exercise, so soldier on.

CHAPTER 9

CHAIR YOGA FOR SENIOR WEIGHT LOSS

With chair yoga, you can shed extra pounds without even standing up. If you have any desire to lose weight or, in any case, maintain your physique, then the following routine is best suited to you.

TARGETING FAT LOSS

There are specific yoga poses that can do a lot for your weight loss ambitions. They are more physically demanding and burn more calories, which is key for weight loss. While they are applicable for weight loss, they can also be used for weight maintenance, i.e., making sure you don't gain any more weight. Remember, though, that exercise is only part of the weight loss journey; your diet is also a large part of what contributes to whether you put on weight or lose it. You can incorporate a day or two of specific weight loss yoga amongst the other days of regular flexibility and mobility yoga. You tailor your yoga experience.

Seated Wide Leg Forward Bend - Seat yourself upright in the chair and spread your legs further than shoulder-width apart, ideally. Spread them out as far as you can without bending your back or straining yourself, and inhale.

Then, you want to place the hands on the knees (initially), and as you start to exhale, you should bend forward from the hips, leaning your chest toward your knees (hinge your body at the hips and fold over).

As you lean forward, move your hands from your knees lower onto your shins and, if you can, all the way until you reach the floor.

Without overexerting yourself, what you want to achieve is to be able to fold far enough ahead that your chest and midsection are flat against your knees.

Seated Spinal Roll - starting in the default seated mountain, relax your arms and let them hang down by your sides with knees at 90-degree bends and feet firmly on the floor.

Start to slowly arch your spine, working through each vertebra.

Then, move to the middle of your back/spine and perform a partial forward fold, where your head and shoulders now move further forward. Finally, work on the lower back, which is leaning even further forward, maintaining that arch in your back as you do so, and finally, be flat on your knees.

After that, you rise; as you do so, arch your back forwards inward to stretch it in the reverse direction and lean back on your chair while you push your shoulders and torso out in front of you to stretch the spine and all those vertebrae one by one.

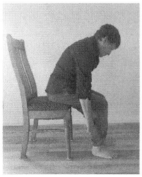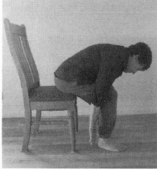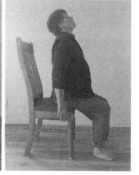

Seated Shoulder Circles - Start in the seated mountain, shoulders relaxed, feet firmly on the ground.

Lift your arms and spread them wide out by your sides, extending them as much as possible and forming a T-pose.

Then, start to slowly rotate your arms in small clockwise, forward circles, feeling the movement in the shoulders.

Keep this up for a while, then reverse the direction of rotation and start making counterclockwise circles.

All the while, your arms should be stretched out at your sides, and your shoulders should rotate with them as you go on.

Seated Alternating Knee-to-Chest - starting from the seated mountain pose, place your hands in your lap, or if additional stability is needed, you can place them on the sides of the chair.

With your back straight and head in line with your torso, lift one knee at a time and bring it towards your chest. If possible, do this without using your hands and simply lift using your back muscles.

If it is not possible, you can place your hands under your knee and pull your knee toward the chest.

After lifting it, you lower it to the floor slowly and switch knees so you are lifting the other knee toward your chest.

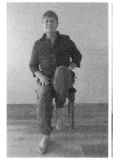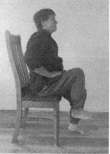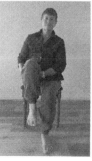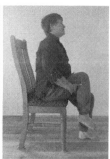

Seated Leg Swings - sit upright in your chair and place your arms on your lap, or if you need additional support, place them by the sides of the chair.

Lift one leg at a time and extend it out in front of you. Ideally, you want there to be no bend in the knees and for you to be able to raise your foot above your hip such that it points upwards.

However, if that is too challenging, you can maintain a slight bend in the knee, and all you have to do is raise the foot to knee level and hold for a little.

Slowly lower your foot back down to the ground, hold for 20 seconds and then lift it again.

Seated Hamstring Stretch - sit upright in the chair and straighten your back. Move forward to the front edge of the chair and stretch out one leg as far forward as you can while keeping it in contact with the floor.

Your heel should be in contact with the floor while your toes are pointed toward the ceiling. Hinge your body at the hips and fold forward slightly.

You should feel some tension in the hamstring of the leg being stretched, hold for 30 seconds.

When done, switch and extend the other leg as well. Do not lean forward too much, as overstretching can injure the muscle.

Keep your back straight, and if you need additional support, hold onto the sides of the chair.

Seated Inner Thigh Stretch - place your upper body in the seated mountain position. Spread your legs wide; as a mini-mum, aim for more than shoulder width apart; ideally, go as wide as you can without injuring your groin.

Then, hinge at the hips and lean forward into the gap created by your open legs.

This should create some pressure and stretching in the inner thighs.

Lean forward as far as you reasonably can, and make sure to hold in a pose where you feel the stretch occurring, hold for 30 seconds.

Once done, rise slowly back into the default seated mountain.

Seated Chest Fly - start in the seated mountain, arms down by your sides and, legs flat on the floor, knees at 90-degree bends.

Then, raise the arms and stretch them out in front of you, touching the palms together. Then separate your palms and pull your arms apart as far as you can; your arms should come to rest stretched out at your sides, leaving you in a T-pose.

If you can, then stretch the arms a little further back to maximise the stretch in your chest muscles.

Hold for 30 seconds, after holding, come back to a resting position where your arms are in front of your chest again.

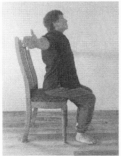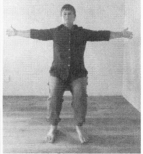

Seated Abdominal Crunches - starting in an upright seated position, place both hands on the sides of the chair you are sitting on.

Move forward so that you are sitting in the middle section of the seat and have some room to lean back.

Using your arms for support, lean backward a little bit, keeping your back straight, and lift both feet off the ground and raise them until there is no bend in the knee and the whole leg to foot is in a straight line.

Lift your legs (simultaneously) and bring them toward your chest while also rising from your leaning position into an upright sitting position.

You should feel a lot of pressure in your core, and your knees do not have to reach your chest; rather, they should come close enough to form a standard V-shape with your torso.

Make sure to move very deliberately as you go through your lifts, and then slowly extend the knees out again and lean back to return to the starting position.

If that is too taxing, you can place your feet on the ground and take a breather between each crunch, although ideally, you carry them out all at once.

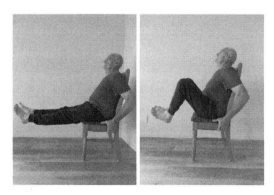

Seated Spinal Twist - Center yourself on the chair and breathe in deep. Raise your arms to about chest height and bend your elbows such that your palms are close to your chest and your elbows are sticking out in either direction (like chicken wings).

You should then turn your upper body - chest, arms, head, etc to one side, keeping your hips firmly planted on the chair.

This stretches the spine, the shoulders, and even the hips and glutes with the crossed leg variation.

If you cannot raise your arms, then place one on your knees and the other behind you, then turn to the side. Hold for thirty seconds, and then repeat three times.

Seated Back Extensions - starting in the seated mountain pose, place your arms down by your sides, gripping the sides of the chair.

Keep your feet flat on the ground and your back straight. Proceed to lengthen your back as much as possible, using your arms for additional support.

You can also tilt your head back a little to maximise the stretch. You should feel some pressure in your back.

Seated Hip Abduction - starting again in the seated mountain pose, place your arms on your lap or on your knees and have your feet firmly on the ground knees at 90-degree bends.

Spread your feet so that they are hip-width apart, and place your palms on the outsides of your knees.

Using your knees, apply pressure and attempt to push them outwards toward your sides while at the same time applying pressure with your hands, resisting that movement.

Hold the position for five seconds and then relax. If you have the equipment, you can use a resistance band and place it just above your knees, and you do not need to use your palms anymore.

Simply try to spread your knees against the force of the resistance bands.

Seated Forward Arm Reach - Seat yourself upright in the chair, arms by your sides and knees at 90 degrees.

Lift your arms and extend them out as far forward as you can while keeping your back straight.

Then, hinge at the hips and fold a little, reaching as far forward as you can with your arms and using them to pull your upper body forward.

You should feel some tension in the upper back, shoulders, and arms.

Seated Triceps Dips -Start in the default seated mountain pose and place your arms on the edges of the seat.

Once done, move forward and sit on the edge of the chair, keeping your arms placed on the sides, knees at 90-degree folds, and feet flat on the ground.

Then you should move your hips completely off the front edge of the chair and support yourself only using your arms; you should then shift your arms so that they hold onto the front lip of the chair while the rest of your body is supported by your arms holding the chair and your legs that are braced by your feet contacting the floor.

Proceed to lower your hips and upper body toward the ground until your elbows are bent at 90 degrees, then stop, hold a little, and rise again, using your arms to lift yourself back up.

For those who feel confident, you should do this exercise with your legs extended as far forward as you can to reduce the amount of support they give your upper body.

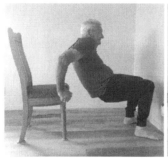
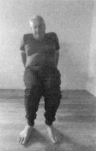

Seated Bridge Pose - Starting with a seated mountain pose, hold the sides of the chair you are sitting on and make sure your feet are firmly placed flat on the ground.

Then, using your arms to support you, lift your hips up off the chair and slowly thrust forward.

Push far out to create a bridge pose, where from your legs up to your head, it should be a smooth, almost convex arch.

In this pose, only go as far out as you can; if you have back issues or knee issues that make this a problem, then do not engage in it.

Frequency, Duration, and Best Workout Tips

It is generally accepted among yoga practitioners and scientists that a decent length for an impactful workout is about 30 to 60 minutes of exercise. This is the general length for workouts targeting improved mobility, balance, coordination, and even weight loss and light endurance.

As a beginner, you should aim to achieve a starting workout time of about 30 minutes. Then, as you go along and build up your endurance and conditioning, you can work out for longer.

Pushing the workout to over 45 minutes and approaching an hour. This is a slow process; do not look to rush it; make sure to prioritise mastering entering and exiting poses correctly, prioritise breathing, and prioritise alignment rather than simply counting the numbers and seconds you worked out.

Like regular exercise, the most important thing is to be consistent with your workouts. Once a week will not cut it, and working out sporadically is also not advised. Set a reasonable schedule where you work out at least four times a week, which can be a mix of some light and more intense workouts on different days. With that, though, be sure to listen to your body. If you are feeling tired or have some pain, take rest days or adjust the workout to avoid aggravating the painful area.

Listening to your body counts during the workouts as well. When a pose is causing pain, ease up on it. Make sure not to overextend or overexert yourself. Quality beats quantity in this business, so a shorter but better-executed workout is better than forcing yourself into an hour-long workout and doing it badly. Worse yet, in doing so, you increase your risk of injury.

As mentioned, consistency is key; working out for 3-5 days is best when looking to maximise the weight loss potential. The relationship between the amount of work and the burning of calories holds, and so theoretically, the more days you do, the more weight you lose (within reason). Yet it is again important to be aware that this process is a slow one and not to rush it too aggressively, hoping to maximise results quickly.

30-40 MINUTE CHAIR YOGA WORKOUT FOR WEIGHT LOSS

Carry out the above-detailed poses and exercises in the below-specified order.

Any yogic breathing technique of choice learned from the previous chapters

Seated Spinal Roll: one minute

Seated Shoulder Circles: two minutes

Seated Alternating Knee-to-Chest: two minutes

Main Workout

Seated Wide Leg Forward Bend: two minutes

Seated Leg Swings: two minutes

Seated Abdominal Crunches: two minutes

Seated Spinal Twist: two minutes

Seated Back Extensions: two minutes

Seated Hip Abduction: two minutes

Seated Forward Arm Reach: two minutes

Seated Triceps Dips: two minutes

Seated Bridge Pose: two minutes

Cool Down

Any meditative pose of choice learned from the previous chapters:

Seated Hamstring Stretch: two minutes

Inner Thigh Stretch: two minutes

Seated Chest Fly: one minute

Tracking Progress

Measure Weight Loss

When looking to exercise regularly, keep an eye on the scale as you carry out your workouts. Measure your weight before you start and carry it out at regular intervals. Keep a journal or notebook where you record your weight loss and other exercise stats. Take photos of yourself to see the visual progress, as well as even take physical measurements such as your waist size, hip width, and thigh width. Again, record these in a journal to track the differences across time. If all goes according to plan, you should see an initial consistent amount of weight loss every two weeks or months, about a pound or even a few, depending on workout intensity and frequency as well as diet. The weight loss will taper off after a while as you reach your optimum weight, where caloric intake matches caloric consumption.

Keeping watch of your physical changes is important as well. Not relating to images and your perception in the mirror. Rather than changes in your overall dimensions. How well do your clothes fit? Are they looser around the waist, around the shoulders, etc.? Maybe you even see some additional muscle definition, and when you flex, they seem a little larger. Keep an eye out for any additional toning from your yoga exercises.

Non-Scale Numeric Victories

Not all gains in the weight loss side of things will necessarily be revealed by the scale and the measuring tape. Do not pin all your expectations on a week-by-week drop in numbers. Other equally beneficial results can be obtained from your exercises. This is especially true if you are close to your optimum weight already.

Keep some attention focused on improvements in your posture, your balance, your coordination, and your mobility. As well as that, keep an eye on your endurance and conditioning. Can you carry out the same poses and hold them for longer without tiring, and can you exercise longer before becoming tired? You will notice that these things start to occur and are positive signs that you are on the right track. If the exercise becomes too easy, then it is an indicator that the intensity needs improving.

The utility of yoga as a weight loss method has been discussed. Next, we will look at Chair Yoga for Pain Relief.

CHAPTER 10

CHAIR YOGA FOR PAIN RELIEF

Pill-free pain relief is possible through chair yoga. A lot of the aches and pains that people experience as they age are usually concentrated in the muscles and joints. Areas which yoga is specifically good for. Through carrying out consistent and uniquely tailored yoga exercises, you can alleviate, if not outright eliminate, most types of physical pain experienced by seniors.

In some instances, pain is hard to treat medically, and the painkillers given do not address the issue directly but only treat the symptoms, which return as soon as the medicine runs out or becomes less effective due to prolonged use. Yoga addresses the cause directly and, if it works, can make a more long-lasting difference. It is free and accessible whenever needed; what you want to achieve is to be able to move freely with no or at least reduced pain. Yoga is a solution that has no side effects is non-addictive, and is only positively impactful on your body and your health.

Each significant and common source of pain in seniors has a series of poses and exercises that specifically target and mobilise that area. This is especially beneficial as it means you can specialise your yoga activities to target the source of your pain more directly. While carrying out the exercises, it is important to be cautious to avoid aggravating the pain when you desire to alleviate it. In general, for significant pain, visit a specialist physician to get an assessment before carrying out any exercises to ensure adverse effects are avoided.

Back Pain Relief

Chair Forward Bend - Seat yourself upright in the chair and spread your legs about shoulder width apart, if not a little further, and inhale.

Then, you want to place the hands on the knees (initially), and as you start to exhale, you should bend forward from the hips, leaning your chest toward your knees. As you lean, move your hands from your knees lower onto your shins and see if you can reach the floor.

Without overexerting yourself, what you want to achieve is to be able to fold far enough ahead that your chest and midsection are flat against your knees.

Chair Upward Salute - Start sitting upright in your chair with your feet flat on the ground, bring your palms together, and place your hands in your lap.

Lift your arms to about head height while keeping palms in contact, engage your lower core and buttocks, and release tension in your back and chest.

Further, raise the arms, but as you do so, arch slightly so you lean more toward one side than the other.

Raise your arms and extend your palms as far out as you can while also arching your body somewhat.

After holding that pose for the determined amount, inhale and stop arching, returning to the centre of the arch in the other direction.

Chair Cat-Cow - place your palms on your legs. You want to let your midsection lean back, pushing the hips and curving the back into a bit of a hunch.

Try to keep your head and shoulders in their initial position (just lowered) while the midsection curls backward, and you push your chest inward (inhaling).

Then come forward and, push your chest out and tilt your head up, arching the back inward toward the thighs and knees (exhaling).

Chair Twist - Center yourself on the chair and breathe in deep. Raise your arms to about chest height and bend your elbows such that your palms are close to your chest and your elbows are sticking out in either direction (like chicken wings).

You should then turn your upper body - chest, arms, head, etc to one side, keeping your hips firmly planted on the chair.

Hold for five breaths, then slowly turn back toward the starting position. Then, repeat in the other direction for a five turns.

Seated Forward Fold - Seat yourself upright in the chair and spread your legs about shoulder width apart, if not a little further, and inhale.

Then, you want to place the hands on the knees (initially), and as you start to exhale, you should bend forward from the hips, leaning your chest toward your knees.

As you lean, move your hands from your knees lower onto your shins and, if you can, keep going until they reach the floor.

Without overexerting yourself, what you want to achieve is to be able to fold far enough ahead that your chest and midsection are essentially flat against your thighs and your hands are firmly on the floor.

Take care not to bend too far forward, as your head should remain on the same level as your knees in the pose's maximum stretch.

Going any further is an advanced technique with different instructions.

Chair Hands-on Knees - this is a relatively simple pose. Starting in the seated mountain, place your palms flat on your knees.

Pushing out using your arms, arch your back outwards, and hunch your shoulders forward.

Stretching your spine. Hold for the specified time, then return to the normal start position.

Benefits

Reduced stiffness

Alleviates back pain

Strengthens back muscles

Larger range of movement

Improved posture

Better sleep quality improved physical capabilities

Neck and Shoulder Tension

Seated Cow - place your palms on your legs. You want to let your midsection lean back, pushing the hips and curving the back into a bit of a hunch. Then come forward and, push your chest out and tilt your head up, arching the back inward toward the thighs and knees (exhaling).

Seated Cat - place your palms on your legs. You want to let your midsection lean back, pushing the hips and curving the back into a bit of a hunch. Try to keep your head and shoulders in their initial position (just lowered) while the midsection curls backward, and you push your chest inward (inhaling).

Chair Neck Stretch - Rock your head side to side and back and forth. Set one side that will be for inhaling, then the opposite side that will be for exhaling.

To do additional stretching, place your hands on the sides of your chair and repeat the process slowly and deliberately. (An alternate exercise is to turn the head to face the left and right directions, turning as far as is comfortable.)

Chair Yoga for Neck and Shoulders Benefits

improved neck stability Released neck tension pain relief improved support to the head

Mental health benefits

Knee and Joint Pain

A way to help you deal with pain in your knees is to stretch and massage them before and after entering into various yoga poses. The stretches and massages are simple and easy to follow but very effective. In a seated position, start by placing the palms under the knee and lifting it off the chair. Then, slowly extend the rest of the lower leg forward as you continue to hold the knees. Extend it, then lower it, and repeat it a few times for each leg. Additionally, you can also massage the knee, raise one foot, and place it across the knee of the other leg. Then, start to slowly move the knee of the foot on top and rock it up and down softly; repeat for a while and then switch knee positions. Placing emphasis on moving the knees in neat circles. Additionally, poses like the warrior I and II, pigeon pose, eagle legs, and others all help stretch the knees as well. The important thing is to be a little more delicate with knee movements while starting out, and as your flexibility and mobility there increases, you can then be more adventurous with your legs.

There are also useful variations that can be adopted to ease the pressure applied on your knees by certain poses, and it is recommended that you avoid exercises and actions that impact the knee while you build up tolerance for it through the stretches and poses. For cardio, avoid fast walking, squatting, single-leg balancing, etc, early on. Look at swimming as a method of cardio that requires less direct input from the knees. Quite quickly, you should feel the pain in your knees start to subside. There is no reason to believe that yoga will magically fix bad joints and so forth, but the symptoms and some of the effects of arthritis and general pain and discomfort can be limited and mitigated.

30-40 MINUTE SENIOR CHAIR YOGA WORKOUT FOR PAIN RELIEF

Warm-up

Any breathing exercises of choice learned from the previous chapters

Neck Stretches - Gently stretch the neck side to side and forward/back to warm up the muscles (30 seconds each)

Shoulder Rolls - When rolling them up and backward, be sure to inhale.

Then exhale as you bring them down and forward.

Repeat the stretch three times. Then, reverse the direction. Inhaling when the chest expands and exhaling when it contracts. Carry out for (30 seconds)

Main Workout

Chair Cat-Cow - Repeat five times.

Seated Forward Bend - Hold for five breaths. Repeat two times.

Chair Twist - Hold for five breaths. Repeat on the left side. Do two sets per side.

Chair Forward Bend - Hold for five breaths. Repeat two times.

Chair Upward Salute - Hold for five breaths. Repeat two times.

Seated Cow - Repeat two times.

Chair Yoga for Knee Pain - Repeat five times for each leg.

Cool Down

Seated Neck Stretch - Hold for 5 breaths. Repeat on the left side.

Seated Forward Fold - Hold for 10 breaths. Close your eyes and take deep breaths (one minute)

Through precise and focused exercises, a lot of the more commonly experienced joint and muscle pain for seniors can be overcome. This is achievable without medication and with no side effects. Additionally, it can be seamlessly incorporated into the rest of the normal exercises carried out by people to maximise the physical and mental gains from yoga exercises.

You know yoga routines for pain relief; you will learn yoga specifically for improving mobility and balance.

CHAPTER 11

TARGETED CHAIR YOGA FOR MOBILITY AND BALANCE

Part of the appeal of yoga is that there is a low barrier to entry, and basically, anyone can carry out most of the major poses. Yet even with that, there are some limitations as to which poses people can do. Some factors are permanent, like significant illness or disability. Yet some of the other constraints, such as bad balance and low mobility, can be overcome through targeted stretches and exercises that, over time, can improve both factors.

This is because balance and mobility are not genetic but rather are developed. This means you can develop the movement and stability you want by working towards it.

HIP OPENER

Tight or immobile hips are a significant challenge to your yoga activity. They reduce your quality of life by limiting your movement and being a potential source of pain. The yoga poses listed below are specifically effective at helping to stretch out and mobilise the hip, lower back, and thigh region of the body.

While results are not guaranteed, there is a high probability that they will be effective at at least mitigating the pain and improving the flexibility and mobility you have in your hips.

Seated Pigeon Pose - In the seated mountain pose, lift one leg and cross it over the other so one leg's ankle rests over the knee of the other.

Hinging at the hips, lean forward with the back still straight so your torso and chest approach your knees. You are essentially forward folding. Keep the hips flat on the chair and then switch to the other leg being crossed over and repeat.

Hold 30 seconds on each side.

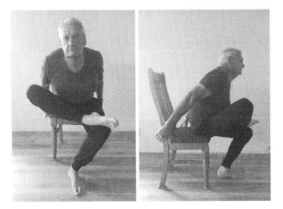

Seated Straddle - position yourself upright in the chair, arms down by your sides, feet on the floor, knees bent at 90 degrees.

Then, move slightly forward on the chair and open your legs wide so that they are no longer in front of you but are on either side of the chair.

Still keeping your back straight, hinge at the hips and fold forward into that gap between your legs.

Go as far forward as you can, ideally folding far enough that your head ends just above the knees, if not even lower down, all the while keeping a straight back.

After holding for 30 seconds, rise again into the upright sitting position and close your legs.

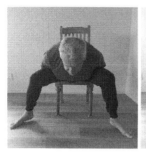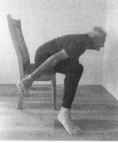

Seated Forward Bend - To maximise this pose, start yourself off in the already explained seated mountain pose.

Back straight, head elevated, feet pushing into the ground. Inhaling into the seated mountain, you then breathe out as you lean forward over your thighs.

In this pose, keep the arms at your sides if you can (keep them on your knees and then lower them to your shins if you need them to support you.)

Bend as far forward as you can without pain and hold that position for five seconds, breathing deeply before coming back to the normal position in the upright seated mountain.

Chair Cat-Cow - Sit upright in your chair with your back straight.

Then, place your palms on your legs. You want to let your midsection lean back, pushing the hips and curving the back into a bit of a hunch.

Try to keep your head and shoulders in their initial position (just lowered) while the midsection curls backward, and you push your chest inward (inhaling).

Then come forward and, push your chest out and tilt your head up, arching the back inward toward the thighs and knees (exhaling).

When you reach the maximum comfortable stretch on each inward/outward stretch, hold the pose for 10 seconds while, then release and slowly engage the other position.

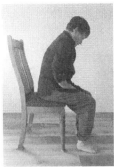 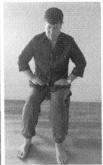 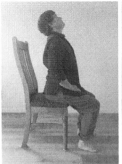 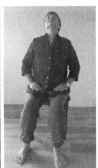

Spinal Twists

Back and spinal tightness causes body-wide side effects. Since the spine is the nerve center and the most significant structural member in the skeleton, any issue with it is a significant hindrance to you. Back pain can result in trouble moving, and even sleeping can be uncomfortable. The yoga poses below are targeted at stretching and easing the muscles and surrounding tissue that encompasses the spine. This is likely to help with, or even prevent, back tightness, spinal problems, and general immobility in that region.

Seated Spinal Twists - for this pose, you will either want a chair without a backrest or, if it's removable, remove it; if you cannot do either, then move forward so you are sitting closer to the edge of your seat.

Again, centre yourself on the chair and breathe in deep. Raise your arms to about chest height and bend your elbows such that your palms are close to your chest. You should then turn your upper body - chest, arms, head, etc to one side, keeping your hips firmly planted on the chair.

Hold for a few breaths, then slowly turn back toward the starting position. Then, repeat in the other direction for a few turns. This exercise stretches the back muscles, the spine, the shoulders, and even the hips and glutes with the crossed leg variation.

Chair Eagle Arms -While seated vertically, fully stretch your arms out in front of you. Then, cross your right hand under and toward the left side of the left arm while still keeping them stretched out in front of you.

The next step is to bend your elbows in both arms to form something close to 90-degree angles pointing upwards. After that, wrap both arms together and, applying most of the force with your right hand, lift your elbows up and simultaneously attempt to drop your shoulders. You should feel some tension and pressure in your arms, shoulders, and upper back.

Hold for five - 10 breaths, then repeat on the other side, simply opposing the order, having your left arm under the right.

Seated Neck Stretches - Rock your head side to side and back and forth. Nice and gentle.

Set one side that will be for inhaling, then the opposite side that will be for inhaling.

To do additional stretching, place your hands on the sides of your chair and repeat the process slowly and deliberately. (An alternate exercise is to turn the head to face the left and right directions, turning as far as is comfortable.)

Arm and Leg Stretches

Arms and legs are the articulating members of the body. They are responsible for carrying out the actual movement that we wish to preserve using yoga. There are instances, though, where, through injury, age, or even just biology, we can have restricted use of these limbs. Trying out some exercises might yield positive results and give you back the freedom of movement you once had in your youth.

Seated Hamstring Stretch - Again, move toward the front edge of your chair. Then, you want to stretch one leg out in front of you as much as you can while keeping your back straight and your head upright.

Then, you want to slowly lean forward, bending at the hips again as you move your chest toward your knees.

Keep doing this until you feel pressure at the back of your thigh, and then hold around that area for a few seconds. You will notice your ability to comfortably bend further forward increasing as time goes on.

Seated Figure Four - Center yourself on the chair with your feet touching the ground.

Then, lift one foot off the ground and place it over the knee to create a figure four with your legs. Keeping your back straight and your hips on the seat, lean forward over your thighs.

Do not arch your back as you lean; remain straight and bend from the hips. You should feel some pressure in the muscles around your hips and lower back, as well as the back of the thigh on the raised leg.

After holding for 20-30 seconds, rise and switch legs, doing the exact same stretch for the same period. Be sure to maintain proper posture and never bounce up and down during the exercise, as it can harm you.

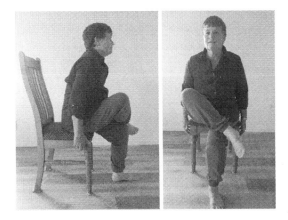

Seated Calf Stretch - For the exercise, you want to sit forward on your chair as much as you can while still being reasonably comfortable.

Then you want to hold onto the sides of your chairs, and, using the muscles in the foot, you want to raise your heels off the ground until you are only being supported by your toes.

Your knees should be elevated above your hips and off the chair completely. Do this as far as you can, aiming at supporting your legs on your tippy toes.

Then hold for a few seconds and then return to normal; in that process, though, rock back onto the soles of your feet, raise your front foot, and try to point your toes toward the ceiling.

After five seconds, return your feet to a flat stance and repeat the process a few times. Throughout both exercises, you should feel tension in your calves.

Seated Chest Expansion - start in the default seated mountain stretch, hands down by the sides. Move your arms out to your sides and inhale as you do. You should feel your chest opening up. If possible, move the arms backward a little as you do so to expand the chest even further. Additionally, you can also lean your head back and push your chest out as far forward as you can without too much strain. Still sitting upright in the chair, you should feel some tension in your chest. Hold for the specified period below, and then lower your arms and reset into the seated mountain pose.

Wrist Stretches - Sit upright and extend one arm out in front of you. With your arm held out in front of you, start to slowly bend your wrist, pointing your hand towards the floor; as that hand is in that position, take your other hand and gently turn the wrist even further down until you feel some pressure in your forearms.

Hold in this position for 20 -30 seconds, and then release and work on the other wrist.Once you have done that, repeat the process of extending your arms and stretching the wrists, but point your hands upwards to the wall in front of you and use the other hand to pull your hand backward until you feel pressure.

For additional stretching, you can also carry out full wrist rolls, where you rotate your hands in 360-degree circles using your wrists. This should be done slowly and deliberately, and it is completely normal to hear a crack or two while doing this.

Another exercise that can accompany this is balling the hands into fists and then un-balling the fists and stretching the fingers.

COMPLETE 30-40 MINUTE SENIOR CHAIR YOGA WORKOUT TO ENHANCE MOBILITY

Implement the above-detailed exercises in the order listed below.

Warm Up

Seated Neck Stretches

Seated Cat Cow

Seating Marching - starting in a basic seated mountain pose with arms by your sides, use your hips and lower back to lift one knee and raise it above the chair and into the air, then quickly lower it and switch and lift the other knee.

Repeat this process quickly in an alternating pattern that resembles marching with high knees. If the exercise is too challenging, a modification to simplify it is to use your arms for bracing by either gripping the sides of the chair while you lift your knees or even using your arms to help lift your knees off the chair and into the air. Do what is within your capabilities.

Seated Wrist Stretches

Main Workout

Seated Butterfly Stretch: orient yourself upright in the chair, back straight, and hands in your lap. Raise your feet off the ground and place them on the front part of the chair.

So it seems as though you have tucked your knees to your chest. After this, spread your knees apart and assume what resembles a cross-legged position but with the soles of your feet making contact with each other.

Then, with this, slowly begin to flap your knees up and down, feeling tension in the inner thighs and, to an extent, the hips.

An easier way to hold the pose is to move forward on your chair and then join the soles of your feet without lifting them off the ground and carry out the exercise from there.

Repeat for 30 seconds.

Seated Pigeon Pose: Hold 30 seconds on each side

Seated Straddle: Hold for 30 seconds

Seated Forward Bend: Hold for 30 seconds

Seated Spinal Twist: 30 seconds on each side

Chair Eagle Arms: 30 seconds on each side

Seated Hamstring Stretch: 30 seconds each leg

Seated Figure Four: 30 seconds on each side

Seated Calf Stretch: 30 seconds each leg

Seated Chest Expansion: Hold for five breaths

Cool Down

Seated Neck RollsSeated Cat-CowSeated ButterflySeated Meditation - Close your eyes and focus on the breath. Hold for one-two minutes.

ACTIVE STEPS

As a senior, look to include other various methods of activity and movement as a way to complement the chair yoga exercises you carry out. This will improve the results you see from your exercises and result in notable benefits such as even further enhanced mobility retention and additional strength and endurance. Some basic exercises are listed below.

Cardio (Walking/Swimming) - remaining active through cardio is one basic but very effective way to ensure you age well. Walking, taking specific care to do so with necessary pumping of the arms, helps with conditioning, balance, and coordination. All of these abilities are in use at the same time while also giving the body a workout. Other methods of cardio are also very effective at maintaining your mobility; cycling is one method, and swimming is another. It is recommended you practice a decent mix of the various cardio types available to you and maximise the benefits of each.

Calf Raises - calf raises are simply standing with your feet flat on the ground. Then, proceed to elevate and stand on your toes, then slowly lower to the ground again, then repeat and lift onto your toes again, and so on. This exercise strengthens the calf muscles, which are important for walking, and even activates muscles in the feet and upper thigh-glute area, which are all essential for balanced movement.

Single Leg Stands/Heel-Toe Walking - standing balanced on a single leg is a good test of whether the strength and balance you have in your leg are still able to carry your weight. Practising it as a workout is a good way to either increase the strength and balance in the leg or to maintain it. The goal should be to successfully balance on one leg for at least a minute, which is something you can work toward. Walking heel to toe is a way to gain extra balance as well since it requires extra coordination to pull off, which will manifest in being better able to maintain balance.

Others - Some suggestions for reasonably achievable and mostly low-impact additional activities are vertical wall push-ups, balancing objects in your hands, rocking the boat, turning side to side, light squats, and many others.

This is to prevent any additional loss of movement in the body as well as to reduce the effects, if not reverse, any that are already being experienced due to aging. The guided exercises in this chapter are important and very useful to further that goal, and especially if you already suffer from diminished movement, try to carry them out.

Having covered the basics of how yoga can improve your movement and balance, you will see an advanced yoga routine to try out.

Chapter 12

Taking it Further: Try An Advanced Workout

This may be the end of this book, but it's just the beginning of your advanced chair yoga journey.

ADVANCED POSES AND HOW TO EXECUTE THEM

Challenging Poses - you can slowly build up the endurance and skill set necessary to carry out the more advanced yoga poses. You can start these poses and hold them for less time than allo- cated here as you work up to it. Focus your first few sessions on safely entering and exiting the poses and making sure your alignment is good.

Flow Sequences -this is basically how well a yoga workout is structured, whether poses link together well into an accessible and efficient workout. A good sequence has poses that comple- ment each other in terms of breathing and activity but that also create seamless movement between exiting one pose and entering the other. Part of flow sequences is determined by your ability to jump between exercises and the endurance to do so consecutively. It will take time to develop a good flow on your end.

Timing and Pace - the pace of yoga should always be slow and deliberate; there is never any need to rush. In regards to time for each stretch, initially aim to hit the specified times in this book, but as you progress and advance, hold the pose for however long you feel you need and you feel is beneficial.

Seated Bound Angle Pose - Sit upright in your chair with your back straight and feet firmly on the floor. Place your palms in your lap and leave them there for now.

Bring your feet together and touch the soles with each other. Then, place your palms on your knees and slightly push them apart a little while keeping a straight back.

If possible, you can raise your legs such that your feet are on the chair as well and you are in a cross-legged position. Then place your palms on your toes and simply use muscles in your legs to lower the knees as much as possible, aiming for them to be flat on the chair at the same level as your hips and toes, or if you can't raise them to chair level add some platform under your feet to elevate them a little while repeating the pose.

Seated Forward Fold with Strap - Execute a normal forward fold as described in previous chapters 6-10, but modify it with the use of a strap attached around the lower thigh, above the knee.

Seated Garland Pose - Start in the default seated mountain position, with arms by the sides. Move forward on the chair and position yourself towards the edge of the seat, moving the feet forward as you do so to ensure the knees retain a 90-degree bend.

Spread the feet slightly wider than hip-width apart and turn the outwards a little so your toes are facing away from each other slightly. Raise your hands up from your sides and toward your chest to touch your palms and form the prayer position.

Then, hinge at the hips and lean forward into the gap that exists between your legs, specifically making sure to place your elbows into the gap created by your legs, having them contact your inner thighs.

Use your legs to push against your elbows as your elbows push against them, and then lean further down. You can additionally lean even further forward to deepen the pose or tuck your feet a little further behind your knees, increasing the bend in the knee. Additionally, you can also place a platform to elevate your feet so that your knees are above your hip level and then carry out the exercise in what resembles a squatting position rather than sitting.

Seated Cow Face Arms - Sit upright in the chair with your back straight and arms by the sides. Move slightly forward of the chair and hold that position.

As you sit, lift one leg and cross it over the other, then move the leg on the bottom inwards a little so your crossed legs are centralized.

Make sure your back is straight as you do this; move your arms so the arm that corresponds with the leg on the top of the cross is touching your shoulder on the same side while the other arm reaches behind you and rests on your lower back.

Then bend your elbows and stretch your arms further, reaching with both hands to try and clasp them together behind your back. Initially, this might be a challenge but stretch as much as you can while keeping a straight back. Ideally, your fingers should make contact in the middle of your back as you are extending from both sides.

When you have achieved that, then push your chest out while holding your arms there and breathe deeply. You should feel pressure in your triceps, your arms, your chest, and especially your hips.

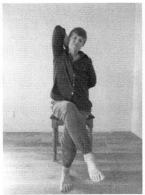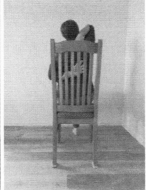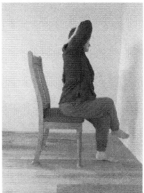

Revolved Half Moon Pose Chair Elbow Block - Start in an upright standing position, this time with your back straight, or as straight as you can manage anyway, stand directly behind the chair.

Place your arms again on the back of the chair to start with. Lift one leg and extend it out behind you and balance on the other leg, holding onto the chair.

Then lean forward and place your elbow on the backrest of the chair, this time using the elbow on the same side as the leg that is raised (you can add some blankets for padding on the backrest, or even place a stable block on there to even the surface out a bit more).

How to achieve this is to turn your torso and head over 90 degrees to face the direction away from where your elbow is. For example, if you raise the right foot, use the right elbow to balance yourself and turn your torso and head toward the left.

Extend the free arms as far upward as you can and hold that pose.

Half Moon Pose With Chair - Starting in an upright standing position, directly behind the chair, you will use the back of the chair as a prop for balance and stability, but this exercise will be done standing.

Place your arms onto the backrest of the chair, as this is what you will use for added stability. Lift one leg up in the air and to the side, only balancing on the other leg and using the chair for stability.

As you do so, lean your body over so your extended leg and torso are in line with each other at an almost horizontal angle. Then hold.

Modifications for Health Conditions

Osteoarthritis

Eagle Pose: Avoid extreme twisting of the knees. Keep the legs crossed gently without forcing the knees. Use light pressure with the arms

Half Moon Pose: Use a chair for support under the hand. Keep the standing leg slightly bent to avoid locking the knee

Diabetes

Seated Forward Bend: Use a strap around the feet to help extend the spine without rounding. Avoid inverting completely

Heart conditions

Seated Forward Bend: Move slowly with control. Avoid straining or holding your breath.

30-40 MINUTE ADVANCED CHAIR YOGA FOR SENIORS

Warm-Up

Any breathing technique of choice learned from the previous chapters

Seated Spinal Roll: hold for one minute

Seated Shoulder Circles: hold for two minutes

Seated Alternating Knee-to-Chest: hold for two minutes

Main Workout

Seated Eagle Pose: Hold for two minutes

Hold the pose for a minute on each side.

Seated Half Moon Pose: hold for two minutes

Hold for a minute on each side.

Seated Bound Angle Pose: hold for two minutes

Seated Forward Fold with Strap: hold for two minutes

Seated Garland Pose: hold for two minutes

Seated Cow Face Arms: two minutes. Hold for a minute on each side.

Revolved Half Moon Pose Chair Elbow Block: two minutes. Hold for a minute on each side.

Half Moon Pose With Chair: two minutes. Hold for a minute on each side.

Cool-Down

Seated Hamstring Stretch: hold for two minutes

Seated Inner Thigh Stretch: hold for two minutes

Seated Chest Fly: hold for one minute

Now that you have learned the makeup of a more advanced yoga routine, you will read about the importance of Modifying Core Chair Yoga Poses for Specific Needs & Objectives.

CHAPTER 13

MODIFYING CORE CHAIR YOGA POSES FOR SPECIFIC NEEDS & OBJECTIVES

No matter your experience or fitness level, you can modify chair yoga poses to align with your goals and personal condition.

CHAIR YOGA WARM-UP POSES AND THEIR SUGGESTED VARIATIONS

Seated Mountain Pose - Sit on a chair with your back straight and your feet firmly planted on the floor - shoulder width apart, rest your palms flat on your thighs.

Then, take a deep breath, extending your spine while simultaneously pushing your feet onto the floor (inhaling). Then, as you start to exhale, draw your stomach in and allow your shoulders to slump a little. As you progress, include turning the head to the left or right direction as you inhale to give the back muscles more of a stretch.

For limited mobility: Do the pose seated in a chair with feet on the floor. Hold onto the sides of the chair for support if needed.

Easier variation: Do the pose with the back against the back of the chair for support. Place hands on the knees instead of at the sides.More difficult: Lift one leg at a time, extending the heel forward while keeping the pose. Repeat five to ten times.

Seated Side Stretch - Reach one arm at a time up over your head toward the ceiling and then lean in the direction opposite where your arm is (Inhaling).

Keep the arm raised and stretched when leaning. Keep the hips firmly placed on the seat.Then, bring the arm down and bring your body out of the lean and back to the vertical position (exhaling) Repeat with each arm in alternate turns 5 times.

For limited mobility: Do the pose while seated in a chair, holding onto the sides for support. Reduce the range of motion of the arch and round.

Easier variation: Place hands on knees instead of the floor to support the back. More difficult: Extend the arms straight in front of you during the cow portion.

Seated Spinal Roll - starting in the default seated mountain, relax your arms and let them hang down by your sides with knees at 90-degree bends and feet firmly on the floor.

Start to slowly arch your spine, working through each vertebra and stretching it. The recommended way to do this is to start with your upper back, lean your head forward, and move your arms lower onto the shins.

Then, move to the middle of your back/spine and perform a partial forward fold, where your head and shoulders now move further forward. Finally, work on the lower back, which is leaning even further forward, maintaining that arch in your back as you do so, and finally, be flat on your knees.

After that, you rise; as you do so, arch your back forward inward to stretch it in the reverse direction and lean back on your chair while you push your shoulders and torso out in front of you to Start in the seated mountain, shoulders relaxed, stretch the spine again, and all those vertebrae one by one.

Repeat for 30 seconds to two minutes.

For limited mobility: Use a smaller range of motion in the roll. Place hands on knees for support.

Easier variation: Roll just the upper back and neck, keeping the lower back stabl e.More difficult: Roll through the entire spine, including the lower back. Extend arms overhead

Seated Shoulder Circles - Start in the seated mountain, shoulders relaxed, feet firmly on the ground.

Lift your arms and spread them wide out by your sides, extending them as much as possible and forming a T-pose.

Then, start to slowly rotate your arms in small clockwise, forward circles, feeling the movement in the shoulders.

Keep this up for a while, then reverse the direction of rotation and start making counterclockwise circles.

All the while, your arms should be stretched out at your sides, and your shoulders should rotate with them as you go on. Repeat for 30 seconds to two minutes.

For limited mobility: Make the circles smaller. Place hands on knees for support.

Easier variation: Do half circles forward and back instead of full circles.More difficult: Straighten arms fully during the circles.

Chair Yoga Flexibility and Stretching Poses and Their Suggested Variations

Seated Forward Fold - Seat yourself upright in the chair and spread your legs about shoulder width apart, if not a little further, and inhale.

Then, you want to place the hands on the knees (initially), and as you start to exhale, you should bend forward from the hips, leaning your chest toward your knees.

As you lean, move your hands from your knees lower onto your shins and see if you can reach the floor. Without overexerting yourself, what you want to achieve is to be able to fold far enough ahead that your chest and midsection are flat against your knees.

Hold for 30 seconds to two minutes.

Easier variation: Sit on the front edge of the chair. Keeping the spine long, hinge slightly forward from the hips. Place hands on shins or thighs. Avoid rounding the spine. Bend the knees slightly if needed.

More difficult variation: Sit on the front edge of the chair. Straighten the legs fully and fold deeper, bringing the chest towards the thighs. Reach arms overhead to deepen the stretch.

Seated Hamstring Stretch - sit upright in the chair and straighten your back. Move forward to the front edge of the chair and stretch out one leg as far forward as you can while keeping it in contact with the floor.

Your heel should be in contact with the floor while your toes are pointed toward the ceiling. Hinge your body at the hips and fold forward slightly.

You should feel some tension in the hamstring of the leg being stretched. When done, switch and extend the other leg as well. Do not lean forward too much, as overstretching can injure the muscle.

Easier variation: Bend one knee, keeping your foot on the floor. Hinge forward from hips over straight leg. Hands can stay on the shin or thigh of the straight leg.

More difficult variation: Straighten the leg completely and flex the foot. Fold deeper, bringing the chest towards the thigh. Reach arms overhead to intensify the stretch.

Seated Inner Thigh Stretch - place your upper body in the seated mountain. Spread your legs wide; as a minimum, aim for more than shoulder width apart; ideally, go as wide as you can without injuring your groin.

Then, hinge at the hips and lean forward into the gap created by your open legs. This should create some pressure and stretching in the inner thighs.

Lean forward as far as you reasonably can, and make sure to hold in a pose where you feel the stretch occurring.

Once done, rise slowly back into the default seated mountain. Hold for 30 seconds to 2 minutes.

Easier variation: Bring soles of feet together, bending knees out to sides if needed. Gently fold forward, keeping the spine long.

More difficult variation: Bring soles of feet together, straightening knees and pressing knees towards the floor. Fold deeply.

Seated Hip Opener - Cross one ankle over the opposite knee. Gently fold forward, keeping the spine long.

More difficult variation: Cross one ankle over the opposite knee, straightening the bottom leg completely. Fold deeply. Hold for 30 seconds to two minutes.

Seated Garland Pose - Bring soles of feet together, knees bent out to sides. Hold onto your ankles.

More difficult variation: Bring soles of feet together, straightening knees and pressing knees down towards the floor. Hold onto your feet. Hold for 30 seconds to two minutes.

Seated Bound Angle Pose - Sit upright in your chair with your back straight and feet firmly on the floor. Place your palms in your lap and leave them there for now.

Bring your feet together and touch the soles with each other. Then, place your palms on your knees and slightly push them apart a little while keeping a straight back.

If possible, you can raise your legs such that your feet are on the chair as well and you are in a cross-legged position.

Then, place your palms on your toes and simply use the muscles in your legs to lower the knees as much as possible, aiming for them to be flat on the chair at the same level as your hips and toes.

Easier variation: Bring soles of feet together, knees bent out to sides. Sit tall.

More difficult variation: Bring soles of feet together, straightening knees and pressing knees down towards the floor. Sit tall

Chair Yoga Strength and Balance Poses and Their Suggested Variations

Seated Warrior I - While in a seated mountain, pose and turn your body to the left side so that your backrest is now on your left.

After that, take your right leg and stick it out behind you, as far back as it can go.

Then, keep your left leg on the chair with a 90-degree bend in the knee, raise your arms above your head, and clasp your palms together.

Limited mobility variation: Sit on the edge of a chair with your right foot flat on the ground and your left leg extended back. Keep your left foot flat on the ground and your left leg straight. Place your hands on your hips.

Easier variation: Keep your left knee bent and your left foot flat on the ground behind you.More difficult variation: Raise your arms overhead, palms facing each other.

Seated Warrior II - Repeat the same procedure as Warrior One, where you stick one leg to the side and then raise your arms.

The difference is that in this pose, you spread your arms out at your sides rather than over your head, and you do not turn to the side but do this one straight on. With arms spread, back straight, and palms down, hold for 30 seconds to two minutes.

Limited mobility variation: Sit sideways on a chair with your right leg bent at a 90-degree angle and your left leg extended straight out to the side. Place your hands on your hips.

Easier variation: Keep your left leg bent and your left foot flat on the ground.M ore difficult variation: Extend your arms out to the sides at shoulder height.

Seated Chair Pose - Start in the seated mountain, with your back straight and your head in line with your torso.

Exhale deeply, and as you do so, lean forward so that your shoulders end up at about halfway along the length of your thighs, which is hard to determine, but you can ballpark it, and as long as it's reasonably close, then it's alright. Next, inhale deeply. As you do so, raise your arms out in front of you, face your palms together, keeping them at shoulder-width distance, then lift them above your head and hold them there as you lean.

Limited mobility variation: Sit on the edge of a chair with your feet hip-width apart and your hands on your thighs.

Easier variation: Keep your hands on your thighs for support.

More difficult variation: Raise your arms overhead, palms facing each other.

Seated Tree Pose - There are multiple variations of the seated tree pose, but a simple one is to sit upright in your chair.

Then again, raise one foot and place it over your knee. Then, bring your arms together into a prayer pose at chest height. You want to inhale while doing this, then exhale as you raise your arms up and above your head.

If you can, you want the arch that is created by your raised arms to be directly overhead, with your arms fully stretched. Hold there for some time, and then lower them to your chest again.

You can then switch which leg is raised and crossing the other.

Limited mobility variation: Sit on a chair with your right foot flat on the ground. Place your left ankle on your right thigh, just above the knee.

Easier variation: Keep your left foot on the ground and your left knee bent.More difficult variation: Raise your arms overhead, palms facing each other.

Seated Half-Moon Pose - Limited mobility variation: Sit on a chair with your feet flat on the ground. Place your left hand on your right knee and your right hand on the back of the chair. Gently twist to the right.

Easier variation: Keep both hands on your knees for support.

More difficult variation: Extend your right arm behind you and your left arm in front of you.

Seated Revolved Half Moon Pose - Limited mobility variation: Sit on a chair with your feet flat on the ground. Place your left hand on your right knee and your right hand on the back of the chair. Gently twist to the right.

Easier variation: Keep both hands on your knees for support.

More difficult variation: Extend your right arm behind you and your left arm in front of you.

Seated Cow Face Arms - Sit upright in the chair with your back straight and arms by the sides. Move slightly forward of the chair and hold that position.

As you sit, lift one leg and cross it over the other, then move the leg on the bottom inwards a little so your crossed legs are centralized. Make sure your back is straight as you do this. To start with, you want to grip the sides of your chair with your hands touching your shoulder on the same side while the other arm reaches behind you and rests on your lower back.

Then bend your elbows and stretch your arms further, reaching with both hands to try and clasp them together behind your back.

Initially, this might be a challenge but stretch as much as you can while keeping a straight back. Ideally, your fingers should make contact in the middle of your back as you are extending from both sides.

When you have achieved that, then push your chest out while holding your arms there and breathe deeply. You should feel pressure in your triceps, in your arms, chest, and especially your hips.

Limited mobility variation: Sit on a chair with your feet flat on the ground. Reach your right arm overhead and bend your elbow, placing your right hand on your upper back. Reach your left arm behind your back and try to clasp your hands together.

Easier variation: Use a strap or towel to bridge the gap between your hands. More difficult variation: Lift your chest and draw your shoulder blades together for a deeper stretch.

Seated Bridge Pose - Starting with a seated mountain pose, hold the sides of the chair you are sitting on and make sure your feet are firmly placed flat on the ground.

Then, using your arms to support you, lift your hips up off the chair and slowly thrust forward. Push far out to create a bridge pose, where from your legs up to your head, it should be a smooth, almost convex arch.

Limited mobility variation: Sit on a chair with your feet flat on the ground and your hands on your hips.

Easier variation: Place your hands on your thighs for support.

More difficult variation: Lift your hips off the chair and extend your arms overhead.

Seated Boat Pose - In this pose, you are again in a seated mountain. To start with, you want to grip the sides of your chair with your hands.

Raise both knees up above the seat into an inclined position and lean back in your chair. Keep your legs suspended in the air without additional support and hold.

Limited mobility variation: Sit on the edge of a chair with your feet flat on the ground. Hold onto the sides of the chair for support.

Easier variation: Keep your feet on the ground and lean back slightly. More difficult variation: Lift your feet off the ground and extend your arms forward.

Chair Yoga Core and Balance Poses and Their Suggested Variations.

Seated Abdominal Crunches - starting in an upright seated position, place both hands on the sides of the chair you are sitting on.

Move forward so that you are sitting in the middle section of the seat and have some room to lean back. Using your arms for support, lean backward a little bit, keeping your back straight, and lift both feet off the ground and raise them until there is no bend in the knee and the whole leg - thigh to foot is in a straight line. Lift your legs (simultaneously) and bring them toward your chest while also rising from your leaning position into an upright sitting position.

You should feel a lot of pressure in your core, and your knees do not have to reach your chest; rather, they should come close enough to form a standard V-shape with your torso. Make sure to move very deliberately as you go through your lifts, and then slowly extend the knees out again and lean back to return to the starting position.

If that is too taxing, you can place your feet on the ground and take a breather between each crunch, although ideally, you carry them out all at once.

Seated Bicycle Crunches - Starting in a seated upright position, be sure to keep your back straight and your feet flat on the ground. Raise your arms and spread them out to your sides, then bend the elbows and bring your hands to rest right beside your head, at about ear height.

Don't hold the head. Simply have the hands located right next to it. Then, start by raising one knee off the floor, bringing it up toward your chest area, and simultaneously bend the back a little and lower the elbow on the opposing side to meet the knee being raised directly in front of your chest.

(Do this without pulling the head at all; simply contort the body independently to make the movements possible). Alternate touching elbow and knee, lower the knee and raise the elbow to their starting position, and switch to the alternate knee elbow pair and do the same. It should resemble a more common set of bicycle crunches but done while sitting.

Chair yoga pain relief and specialised poses and their suggested variations

Seated Spinal Twist - Center yourself on the chair and breathe in deep. Raise your arms to about chest height and bend your elbows such that your palms are close to your chest and your elbows are sticking out in either direction (like chicken wings).

You should then turn your upper body - chest, arms, head, etc to one side, keeping your hips firmly planted on the chair.

Hold for a few breaths, then slowly turn back toward the starting position. Then, repeat in the other direction for a few turns.

This exercise stretches the back muscles, the spine, the shoulders, and even the hips and glutes with the crossed leg variation.

If you cannot raise your arms, then place one on your knees and the other behind you, then turn to the side.

Seated Back Extensions - starting in the seated mountain pose, place your arms down by your sides, gripping the sides of the chair.

Keep your feet flat on the ground and your back straight. Proceed to lengthen your back as much as possible, using your arms for additional support. You can also tilt your head back a little to maximise the stretch. You should feel some pressure in your back.

Seated Hip Abduction - starting again in the seated mountain, place your arms on your lap or on your knees and have your feet firmly on the ground knees at 90-degree bends.

Spread your feet so that they are hip-width apart, and place your palms on the outsides of your knees.

Using your knees, apply pressure and attempt to push them outwards toward your sides while at the same time applying pressure with your hands, resisting that movement.

Hold the position for five seconds and then relax. If you have the equipment, you can use a resistance band and place it just above your knees, and you do not need to use your palms anymore.

Simply try to spread your knees against the force of the resistance bands.

Seated Forward/Upward Arm Reach - Seat yourself upright in the chair, arms by your sides and knees at 90 degrees.

Lift your arms and extend them out as far forward as you can while keeping your back straight.

Then, hinge at the hips and fold a little, reaching as far forward as you can with your arms and using them to pull your upper body forward.

You should feel some tension in the upper back, shoulders, and arms.

Seated Triceps Dips - Start in the default seated mountain pose and place your arms on the edges of the seat.

Once done, move forward and sit on the edge of the chair, keeping your arms placed on the sides, knees at 90-degree folds, and feet flat on the ground.

Then you should move your hips completely off the front edge of the chair and support yourself only using your arms; you should then shift your arms so that they hold onto the front lip of the chair while the rest of your body is supported by your arms holding the chair and your legs that are braced by your feet contacting the floor.

Proceed to lower your hips and upper body toward the ground until your elbows are bent at 90 degrees, then stop, hold a little, and rise again, using your arms to lift yourself back up.

Seated Revolved Half Moon Pose Chair Elbow Block - Starting in an upright standing position, this time with your back straight, or as straight as you can manage anyway, stand directly behind the chair.

Place your arms again on the back of the chair to start with. Lift one leg and extend it out behind you and balance on the other leg, holding onto the chair.

Then lean forward and place your elbow on the backrest of the chair, this time using the elbow on the same side as the leg that is raised (you can add some blankets for padding on the backrest, or even place a stable block on there to even the surface out a bit more).

How to achieve this is to turn your torso and head over 90 degrees to face the direction away from where your elbow is. For example, if you raise the right foot, use the right elbow to balance yourself and turn your torso and head toward the left.

Extend the free arms as far upward as you can and hold that pose.

Half Moon Pose with Chair - Starting in an upright standing position, directly behind the chair. This time, you will use the back of the chair as a prop for balance and stability, but this exercise will be done standing.

Place your arms onto the backrest of the chair, as this is what you will use for added stability. Lift one leg up in the air and to the side, only balancing on the other leg and using the chair for stability.

As you do so, lean your body over so your extended leg and torso are in line with each other at an almost horizontal angle. Then hold.

Chair Yoga Relaxation and Cool-Down Poses and Their Suggested Variations

Seated Savasana - Before starting, move your chair and place it directly in front of a wall such that as you sit down, you have the wall immediately behind you.

Then take your seat in the chair, assuming the seated mountain, back straight and feet on the ground. With the legs shoulder width apart, you can use a prop that you place between your thighs to maintain that distance.

Then you want to lean the head back slightly, tilt the face upward just a little bit, and place your hands, palms facing upward on your thighs, and let them rest there. Hold this pose.

Seated Meditation Pose - sit upright in your chair, either place your hands flat on your thighs, palms up, or in the prayer position in front of your chest.

Seated Chest Fly - start in the seated mountain, arms down by your sides and, legs flat on the floor, knees at 90-degree bends.

Then, raise the arms and stretch them out in front of you, touching the palms together.

Then separate your palms and pull your arms apart as far as you can; your arms should come to rest stretched out at your sides, leaving you in a T-pose.

If you can, then stretch the arms a little further back to maximise the stretch in your chest muscles.

After holding, come back to a resting position where your arms are in front of your chest again.

Seated Alternating Knee-to-Chest - starting from the seated mountain pose, place your arms on your lap, or if additional stability is needed, you can place them on the sides of the chair.

With your back straight and head in line with your torso, lift one knee at a time and bring it towards your chest. If possible, do this without using your hands and simply lift using your back muscles.

If it is not possible, you can place your hands under your knee and pull your knee toward the chest.

After lifting it, you need additional support. Lower it to the floor slowly and switch knees so you are lifting the other knee toward your chest.

Seated Leg Swings - sit upright in your chair and place your arms on your lap, or if you need additional support, place them by the sides of the chair.

Lift one leg at a time and extend it out in front of you. Ideally, you want there to be no bend in the knees and for you to be able to raise your foot above your hip such that it points upwards.

However, if that is too challenging, you can maintain a slight bend in the knee, and all you have to do is raise the foot to knee level and hold for a little.

Slowly lower your foot back down to the ground, hold for a little and then lift it again.

Basic How to Modify the Core Chair Yoga Poses to Fit Your Goal and Condition

Some general rules to observe when carrying out the poses and looking to make them as impactful as possible while also respecting that you aren't as mobile is to reduce the range of motion. Especially when starting out, it is common for the necessary flexibility to be lacking, so do not force it.

Additionally, listen to your body; when it communicates to you through discomfort and pain, those are signals that you should ease up or stop entirely. Part of what you can do is to also use props and comfort accessories, blankets, blocks, bands, and so on, which can be used in a variety of creative ways to make exercises more achievable and practical for those with limited mobility.

For those who find that the poses are a little too easy, there is also work you can do, which is to make exercises even harder for yourself. The big thing is to increase the range of motion (within reason) to stretch and strengthen the muscles further. There is a limit to this, though; forcing extra movement from a stretch past a certain point can disturb alignment and cause injury, as well as produce limited results. Not making use of props as well, allowing the body to support itself, and holding poses for longer all contribute to making the pose harder for you overall.

7 Day Fitness Program

Welcome to your 7-day Chair Yoga journey! You're about to embark on a wonderful adventure that will gently guide you towards improved flexibility, strength, balance, and overall well-being. Chair Yoga is a fantastic way to stay active and maintain your independence, all from the comfort of your chair. Remember, each small step you take is a powerful move towards a healthier and happier you.

Embrace this time for yourself, listen to your body, and enjoy the process. You've made a great choice, and we're here to support you every step of the way. Let's get started on this empowering journey together!

This program starts with 10 minutes daily and gradually builds up to 15 minutes daily. The exercises are gentle and focus on balance, flexibility and stability. If needed adjust the exercises to match your fitness level. Always listen to your body and consult with a healthcare professional before starting any new exercise program.

Day 1: Introduction and Gentle Warm-Up (10 minutes)

Warm-Up (2 minutes)

- **Seated Shoulder Rolls:** Sit comfortably in a chair with your feet flat on the floor. Slowly roll your shoulders forward and backward for one minute.

- **Gentle Neck Stretches:** Sit comfortably in a chair and gently tilt your head towards one shoulder, hold for five seconds, and repeat on the other side for one minute.

Chair Yoga Exercises (6 minutes)

- **Seated Cat-Cow:** Sit on a chair with your feet flat on the floor and hands on your knees. Arch your back and look up (Cow), then round your back and tuck your chin (Cat), do this motion for two minutes.

- **Seated Forward Bend:** Sit on a chair with your feet flat on the floor and gently bend forward from the hips, reaching towards your toes, hold this position for 30 seconds and repeat four times.

- **Seated Spinal Twist:** Sit on a chair with your feet flat on the floor, place your right hand on the back of the chair, and twist to the right. Hold for 30 seconds, then switch sides and hold for 30 seconds.

- **Seated Knee Lifts:** Sit on a chair with your feet flat on the floor and lift one knee towards your chest, hold for 30 seconds, then lower it back down. Repeat with the other leg holding for 30 seconds.

Cool Down (2 minutes)

- **Gentle Breathing:** 2 minutes

Day 2: Core and Stability (10 minutes)

Warm-Up (2 minutes)

- **Seated Marching:** Sit on a chair with your feet flat on the floor and lift your knees alternately as if marching for one minute.

- **Gentle Side Bends:** Sit on a chair with your feet flat on the floor. Gently bend to one side, reaching your arm over your head, hold for 30 seconds, then repeat on the other side.

Chair Yoga Exercises (6 minutes)

- **Seated Sun Salutation:** Sit on a chair with your feet flat on the floor and arms by your sides. Raise your arms overhead, bend forward, hold for 30 seconds, and return to the starting position. Repeat four times.

- **Seated Leg Extensions:** Sit on a chair with your feet flat on the floor and extend one leg out straight, hold for 30 seconds, then lower it back down. Repeat with the other leg.

- **Seated Shoulder Stretch:** Sit on a chair with your feet flat on the floor and extend one arm out in front of you, using the other arm to gently put it across your chest, hold this position for 30 seconds. Switch arms. Repeat this four times.

- **Seated Hip Opener:** Sit on a chair with your feet flat on the floor, place one ankle on the opposite knee, and gently press down on the knee for a hip stretch hold for 30 seconds, and repeat on the other side.

Cool Down (2 minutes)

- **Gentle Breathing:** 2 minutes

Day 3: Flexibility and Range of Motion (12 minutes)

Warm-Up (2 minutes)

- **Seated Arm Circles:** Sit on a chair with your feet flat on the floor and extend your arms to the sides. Make small circles with your arms for one minute.

- **Gentle Leg Swings:** Sit on a chair with your feet flat on the floor and gently swing one leg forward and backward for 30 seconds. Repeat with the other leg.

Chair Yoga Exercises (8 minutes)

- **Seated Side Stretch:** Sit on a chair with your feet flat on the floor and reach one arm, bend it over your head to the other side hold for 30 seconds, then switch sides. Repeat this four times.

- **Seated Hamstring Stretch:** Sit on a chair with one leg extended straight out at knee height pointing your toes back towards your body, hold for 30 seconds and switch legs. Repeat this four times.

- **Seated Ankle Rotations:** Sit on a chair with your feet flat on the floor and lift one foot off the ground. Rotate your ankle in circles for 30 seconds, and switch ankles. Repeat four times.

- **Seated Chest Opener:** Sit on a chair with your feet flat on the floor and clasp your hands behind your back. Lift your hands slightly and open your chest. Hold for 30 seconds, then come back to the resting position. Repeat four times.

Cool Down (2 minutes)

- **Deep Breathing:** 2 minutes

Day 4: Strength and Conditioning (12 minutes)

Warm-Up (2 minutes)

- **Seated Gentle Walking in Place:** Sit on your chair and move your feet as if walking in place for one minute.

- **Seated Shoulder Shrugs:** Sit on your chair with your feet flat on the floor and lift your shoulders towards your ears, then lower them back down for one minute.

Chair Yoga Exercises (8 minutes)

- **Seated Warrior I:** Sit on your chair with your feet flat on the floor, extend one leg to the side, and reach your arms overhead. Hold for 30 seconds, then switch sides. Repeat four times.

- **Seated Warrior II:** Sit on your chair with your feet flat on the floor, extend one leg to the side, and reach your arms out to the sides. Hold for 30 seconds, then switch sides. Repeat four times.

- **Seated Chair Pose:** Sit on your chair with your feet flat on the floor and extend your arms overhead. Engage your core and hold for 30 seconds. Repeat four times.

- **Seated Side Plank:** Sit sideways in the chair, place one forearm on the seat, and lift your body to form a side plank. Hold for 30 seconds, then switch sides. Repeat two times on each side.

Cool Down (2 minutes)

- **Gentle Stretching:** 2 minutes

Day 5: Rest and Recovery (10 minutes)

Gentle Activity

- **Relaxed Seated Breathing:** Sit comfortably and focus on deep, slow breaths for five minutes.

- **Light-Seated Stretching:** Perform gentle stretches of your choice for the whole body while seated for five minutes.

Day 6: Balance and Coordination (15 minutes)

Warm-Up (3 minutes)

- **Seated Gentle Leg Swings:** Sit on your chair with your feet flat on the floor gently swing one leg at a time in front of you holding your core for 1.5 minutes.

* **Seated Arm Circles:** Sit on your chair with your feet flat on the floor and extend your arms to the sides. Make small circles with your arms for 1.5 minutes.

Chair Yoga Exercises (10 minutes)

* **Seated Toe Taps:** Sit on your chair with your feet flat on the floor and tap your toes on the ground alternately for 2.5 minutes.

* **Seated Marching:** Sit on your chair with your feet flat on the floor and lift your knees alternately as if marching for 2.5 minutes.

* **Seated Heel Raises:** Sit on your chair with your feet flat on the floor and lift your heels off the ground, then lower them back down for 2.5 minutes.

* **Seated Figure-8 Arms:** Sit on your chair with your feet flat on the floor and extend your arms. Move them in a figure-8 pattern for 2.5 minutes.

Cool Down (2 minutes)

* **Gentle Leg and Arm Stretches:** 2 minutes

Day 7: Full Body Integration (15 minutes)

Warm-Up (3 minutes)

* **Seated Gentle Jogging in Place:** Sit on your chair and move your legs as if jogging in place for 1.5 minutes.

* **Seated Arm Circles:** Sit on your chair with your feet flat on the floor and extend your arms to the sides. Make small circles with your arms for 1.5 minutes

Chair Yoga Exercises (10 minutes)

- **Seated Sun Salutation:** Sit on a chair with your feet flat on the floor and arms by your sides. Raise your arms overhead, bend forward, hold for 30 seconds, and return to the starting position. Repeat five times.

- **Seated Cat-Cow:** Sit on a chair with your feet flat on the floor and hands on your knees. Arch your back and look up (Cow), then round your back and tuck your chin (Cat), do this motion for 2.5 minutes.

- **Seated Forward Bend:** Sit on a chair with your feet flat on the floor and gently bend forward from the hips, reaching towards your toes, hold this position for 30 seconds and repeat five times.

- **Seated Spinal Twist:** Sit on a chair with your feet flat on the floor, place your right hand on the back of the chair, and twist to the right. Hold for 30 seconds, then switch sides and hold for 30 seconds. Repeat for 2.5 minutes.

Cool Down (2 minutes)

- **Gentle Full Body Stretch:** 2 minutes

Congratulations on completing the 7-day Chair Yoga program! Your dedication and commitment to improving your health and well-being are truly commendable.

By focusing on flexibility, strength, balance, and mindfulness, you've taken significant steps toward enhancing your overall fitness and quality of life. Remember, this is just the beginning of your journey.

Continue to incorporate these gentle yet effective exercises into your daily routine to maintain and build upon the progress you've made. Celebrate your achievement and know that each day of practice brings you closer to a healthier, happier you. Well done!

Now you've mastered the 7-Day Program, move on to the next chapter – the 28-Day Program.

28 Day Fitness Program

Embarking on a 28-day Chair Yoga fitness program is a wonderful step towards enhancing your health and well-being. This gentle and accessible practice is designed to improve your strength, flexibility, and relaxation. Remember, every journey begins with a single step, and by committing to this program, you are prioritising your health and investing in a brighter, more active future. Stay positive, be patient with yourself, and enjoy the process. You've got this!

This program starts with 10 minutes a day and gradually builds up to 20 minutes per day. The exercises are gentle and designed to improve strength, flexibility, and relaxation.

Adjust the exercises as needed to match your fitness level and comfort. Always listen to your body and consult with a healthcare professional before starting any new exercise program.

Week 1: Introduction (10 minutes/day)

Day 1-2:

1. **Seated Mountain Pose** - 1 minute

2. **Seated Cat-Cow Stretch** - 2 minutes

3. **Seated Forward Bend** - 2 minutes

4. **Seated Side Stretch** - 2 minutes (1 minute each side)

5. **Seated Spinal Twist** - 3 minutes (1.5 minutes each side)

Day 3:

- Rest Day

Day 4-5:

1. **Seated Mountain Pose** - 1 minute

2. **Seated Cat-Cow Stretch** - 2 minutes

3. **Seated Forward Bend** - 2 minutes

4. **Seated Side Stretch** - 2 minutes (1 minute each side)

5. **Seated Spinal Twist** - 3 minutes (1.5 minutes each side)

Day 6:

1. **Seated Mountain Pose** - 1 minute

2. **Seated Cat-Cow Stretch** - 2 minutes

3. **Seated Forward Bend** - 2 minutes

4. **Seated Side Stretch** - 2 minutes (1 minute each side)

5. **Seated Spinal Twist** - 3 minutes (1.5 minutes each side)

Day 7:

- Rest Day

Week 2: Building Strength (12 minutes/day)

Day 8-9:

1. **Seated Mountain Pose** - 1 minute

2. **Seated Cat-Cow Stretch** - 2 minutes

3. **Seated Forward Bend** - 2 minutes

4. **Seated Side Stretch** - 2 minutes (1 minute each side)

5. **Seated Spinal Twist** - 3 minutes (1.5 minutes each side)

6. **Seated Leg Lifts** - 2 minutes (1 minute each leg)

Day 10:

- Rest Day

Day 11-12:

1. **Seated Mountain Pose** - 1 minute

2. **Seated Cat-Cow Stretch** - 2 minutes

3. **Seated Forward Bend** - 2 minutes

4. **Seated Side Stretch** - 2 minutes (1 minute each side)

5. **Seated Spinal Twist** - 3 minutes (1.5 minutes each side)

6. **Seated Leg Lifts** - 2 minutes (1 minute each leg)

Day 13:

1. **Seated Mountain Pose** - 1 minute

2. **Seated Cat-Cow Stretch** - 2 minutes

3. **Seated Forward Bend** - 2 minutes

4. **Seated Side Stretch** - 2 minutes (1 minute each side)

5. **Seated Spinal Twist** - 3 minutes (1.5 minutes each side)

6. **Seated Leg Lifts** - 2 minutes (1 minute each leg)

Day 14:

- Rest Day

Week 3: Adding Variety (15 minutes/day)

Day 15-16:

1. **Seated Mountain Pose** - 1 minute

2. **Seated Cat-Cow Stretch** - 2 minutes

3. **Seated Forward Bend** - 2 minutes

4. **Seated Side Stretch** - 2 minutes (1 minute each side)

5. **Seated Spinal Twist** - 3 minutes (1.5 minutes each side)

6. **Seated Leg Lifts** - 2 minutes (1 minute each leg)

7. **Seated Shoulder Rolls** - 3 minutes (1.5 minutes each direction)

Day 17:

- Rest Day

Day 18-19:

1. **Seated Mountain Pose** - 1 minute

2. **Seated Cat-Cow Stretch** - 2 minutes

3. **Seated Forward Bend** - 2 minutes

4. **Seated Side Stretch** - 2 minutes (1 minute each side)

5. **Seated Spinal Twist** - 3 minutes (1.5 minutes each side)

6. **Seated Leg Lifts** - 2 minutes (1 minute each leg)

7. **Seated Shoulder Rolls** - 3 minutes (1.5 minutes each direction)

Day 20:

1. **Seated Mountain Pose** - 1 minute

2. **Seated Cat-Cow Stretch** - 2 minutes

3. **Seated Forward Bend** - 2 minutes

4. **Seated Side Stretch** - 2 minutes (1 minute each side)

5. **Seated Spinal Twist** - 3 minutes (1.5 minutes each side)

6. **Seated Leg Lifts** - 2 minutes (1 minute each leg)

7. **Seated Shoulder Rolls** - 3 minutes (1.5 minutes each direction)

Day 21:

- Rest Day

Week 4: Building Endurance (20 minutes/day)

Day 22-23:

1. **Seated Mountain Pose** - 1 minute

2. **Seated Cat-Cow Stretch** - 2 minutes

3. **Seated Forward Bend** - 2 minutes

4. **Seated Side Stretch** - 2 minutes (1 minute each side)

5. **Seated Spinal Twist** - 3 minutes (1.5 minutes each side)

6. **Seated Leg Lifts** - 2 minutes (1 minute each leg)

7. **Seated Shoulder Rolls** - 3 minutes (1.5 minutes each direction)

8. **Seated Ankle Rolls** - 3 minutes (1.5 minutes each foot)

9. **Seated Chest Opener** - 2 minutes

Day 24:

- Rest Day

Day 25-26:

1. **Seated Mountain Pose** - 1 minute

2. **Seated Cat-Cow Stretch** - 2 minutes

3. **Seated Forward Bend** - 2 minutes

4. **Seated Side Stretch** - 2 minutes (1 minute each side)

5. **Seated Spinal Twist** - 3 minutes (1.5 minutes each side)

6. **Seated Leg Lifts** - 2 minutes (1 minute each leg)

7. **Seated Shoulder Rolls** - 3 minutes (1.5 minutes each direction)

8. **Seated Ankle Rolls** - 3 minutes (1.5 minutes each foot)

9. **Seated Chest Opener** - 2 minutes

Day 27:

1. **Seated Mountain Pose** - 1 minute

2. **Seated Cat-Cow Stretch** - 2 minutes

3. **Seated Forward Bend** - 2 minutes

4. **Seated Side Stretch** - 2 minutes (1 minute each side)

5. **Seated Spinal Twist** - 3 minutes (1.5 minutes each side)

6. **Seated Leg Lifts** - 2 minutes (1 minute each leg)

7. **Seated Shoulder Rolls** - 3 minutes (1.5 minutes each direction)

8. **Seated Ankle Rolls** - 3 minutes (1.5 minutes each foot)

9. **Seated Chest Opener** - 2 minutes

Day 28:

- Rest Day

Exercise Descriptions

1. **Seated Mountain Pose:** Sit tall in your chair with your feet flat on the floor, hands resting on your thighs. Focus on your breath and hold this posture.

2. **Seated Cat-Cow Stretch:** Sit on the edge of the chair, place your hands on your knees. Inhale, arch your back and look up (Cow). Exhale, round your back and tuck your chin to your chest (Cat).

3. **Seated Forward Bend:** Sit tall and hinge forward at your hips, reaching your hands towards the floor or your ankles.

4. **Seated Side Stretch:** Sit tall, place one hand on the chair seat, and reach the other arm up and over your head, stretching to the side.

5. **Seated Spinal Twist:** Sit tall, place one hand on the opposite knee, and gently twist your torso, looking over your shoulder. Repeat on the other

side.

6. **Seated Leg Lifts:** Sit tall, lift one leg straight out in front of you, hold for a few seconds, then lower it back down. Repeat with the other leg.

7. **Seated Shoulder Rolls:** Sit tall, roll your shoulders up, back, and down in a circular motion.

8. **Seated Ankle Rolls:** Sit tall, lift one foot off the floor and roll your ankle in a circular motion. Repeat with the other foot.

9. **Seated Chest Opener:** Sit tall, interlace your fingers behind your back, and gently lift your hands to open your chest.

Congratulations on reaching the end of your 28-day Chair Yoga journey! Your dedication and perseverance have paid off, and you've successfully embraced a routine that promotes strength, flexibility, and overall well-being.

It's no small feat to commit to a month-long program, and your commitment to enhancing your health and vitality is truly commendable. May this milestone inspire you to continue incorporating gentle and effective practices into your daily life. Well done!

Conclusion

While the book is over, your journey will continue; with all you have learned and the loads more you will come to learn about chair yoga, try to maximise the utility you get out of its benefits. If you have limited mobility that has improved, be more active and go out; do more for yourself. Age shouldn't be a limiting factor, and with a body kept in shape through yoga, you can give yourself the freedom and ability to do whatever you please.

Go through the exercises at a calm pace, focusing mostly on achieving the right alignment and mastery of the poses to ensure sustainable long-term benefit. Through easy-to-follow chair yoga exercises that you can do at home, you can unlock a healthier, happier, and more independent life throughout your senior years.

The only real necessity to success with chair yoga is determination and consistency; everything else can and will be learned. The essence of this book is empowerment – empowerment to transform the quality of your senior years, maintain personal independence for as long as possible, and enjoy all the things you have always enjoyed in life, even as you advance in age. Go ahead and live a fulfilling and enriching life with family, friends, and your community. If you can, try to make a difference in the lives of others and either teach them the basics of yoga yourself or recommend this book to them so they also start to experience the life-altering benefits that chair yoga brings.

Make chair yoga a daily habit and turn your golden years into your best years. Start with the beginner routine and watch your life transform, one pose at a time.

MAKE A DIFFERENCE WITH YOUR REVIEW

If you found this book helpful, informative, or useful, then please do leave a review on Google or Amazon, as it helps get this book out to more people who can also benefit just as you did.

Now you have everything you need to find relief, balance, and independence, it's time to pass on your newfound knowledge and show other readers where they can find the same help.

Simply by leaving your honest opinion of this book on Amazon, you'll show other seniors where they can find the information they're looking for and pass their passion for chair yoga forward.

Thank you for your help. The practice of chair yoga for seniors is kept alive when we pass on our knowledge – and you're helping me to do just that.

Your review can make a difference for someone who's on the fence about starting their journey into chair yoga. Share your thoughts and let them know how this book has impacted your life.

Remember, your experiences and insights can be the guiding light for others seeking the benefits of chair yoga.

Thank you once again for being a part of this journey and for sharing the love of chair yoga with others.

Your biggest fan, Laurel Harris

Scan the QR code to leave your review!

OTHER BOOKS IN THE SERIES

Thank you so much for joining me on this journey through Chair Yoga & Wall Pilates for Seniors.

If you are interested in any other books in the Fitness and Self Help for Seniors Series please check out my other books below – thank you.

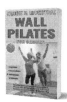

REFERENCES

8 foods older adults should avoid eating. (n.d.). Sun Health Communities. https:// www.sunhealthcommunities.org/helpful-tools/articles/8-foods-o lder- adults-avoid-eating

9 Yogic Breathing Practices for Mind-Body Balance and Healing. (n.d.) . https://www. himalayanyogainstitute.com/9-yogic-breathing-practices-mind -body- balance-healing/

10 yoga poses you can do sitting in a chair. (2023, August 25). TODAY.com. https:// www.today.com/health/diet-fitness/chair-yoga-poses-rcna101778

350+ Chair Yoga poses to Plan yoga sequences | Tummee.com. (n.d.). https://www. tummee.com/yoga-poses/chair-yoga-poses

Anthony. (2018, October 16). *5 simple reasons people choose chair yoga for exercise - My senior Health plan*. My Senior Health Plan. https://www.myseniorhealth plan.com/blog/2018/10/16/5-reasons-people-choose-chair-yoga/

Ardentwhiddonmain. (2023a, June 2). *The Mental Health Benefits of Exercise For Older Adults | Whiddon*. YourLife. https://www.whiddon.com.au/yourlife/the-mental-health-benefits-of-exercise-for-older-adults/

Ardentwhiddonmain. (2023b, June 2). *The Mental Health Benefits of Exercise For Older Adults | Whiddon*. YourLife. https://www.whiddon.com.au/yourlife/the-mental-health-benefits-of-exercise-for-older-adults/

Benedetti, M. G., Furlini, G., Zati, A., & Mauro, G. L. (2018). The effectiveness of physical exercise on bone density in osteoporotic patients. *BioMed Research International*, *2018*, 1–10. https://doi.org/10.1155/2018/4840531

Blissability Accessible Yoga. (2021, February 21). *Accessible Chair Yoga: 5 minute breathing & stretching* [Video]. YouTube. https://www.youtube.com/watch?v=4iwJPyOAw4g

Bottoms Down. (2021, January 28). *Chair yoga - weight loss - 30 minutes some seated, more standing* [Video]. YouTube. https://www.youtube.com/watch? v=ZEoJD7OCZtg

Bottoms Down. (2023a, February 22). *Chair Yoga - Weight Loss with Therese - 30 Minutes Seated* [Video]. YouTube. https://www.youtube.com/watch?v=53AarSZGcvY

Bottoms Down. (2023b, February 22). *Chair Yoga - Weight Loss with Therese - 30 Minutes Seated* [Video]. YouTube. https://www.youtube.com/watch?v=53AarSZGcvY

Branding, A. (n.d.). Arad Branding. *Arad Branding*. https://aradbranding.com/en/chair-yoga-for-seniors-poses-ball/

Brandy, B. (2022, January 19). *Great Benefits Of Chair Yoga For Seniors*. Aston Gardens. https://www.astongardens.com/senior-living-blog/great-benefits-of-chair-yoga-for-seniors/

Breath, M. (2020, July 19). *Four Chair Yoga poses to release tight shoulders, neck and back*. Mindfulness Course Singapore. https://mindfulbreath.sg/four-chair-yoga-poses-to-release-tight-shoulders-neck-and-back-mindfulbreath-y/

Carolann Rose Yoga. (2021, May 11). *30 minute Chair Yoga | Intermediate Chair Yoga | Carolann Rose Yoga* [Video]. YouTube. https://www.youtube.com/watch?v=aVB4bM0kas4

Center Space Yoga. (2022, August 2). *Chair Yoga hip stretches for beginners, Seniors, and EveryBody: 15 minutes* [Video]. YouTube. https://www.youtube.com/ watch?v=MDDZp-YkDmA

Chair neck stretch yoga | Yoga sequences, benefits, variations, and Sanskrit pronuncia- tion | Tummee.com. (2019, February 12). Tummee.com. https://www.tummee. com/yoga-poses/chair-neck-stretch

Chair Seated Warm Up Flow Yoga | Yoga Sequences, Benefits, Variations, and Sanskrit Pronunciation | Tummee.com. (2019, July 15). Tummee.com. https://www.tummee.com/yoga-poses/chair-seated-warm-up-flow

Chair Yoga and Why Seated Yoga Poses Are Good For You | Lifespan. (n.d.) . Lifespan. https://www.lifespan.org/lifespan-living/chair-yoga-and-why-seated -yoga- poses-are-good-you

Chair Yoga Poses | How to get started with chair yoga. (n.d.). Chair Yoga Poses | How to Get Started With Chair Yoga. https://www.uaex.uada.edu/life-skills-w ell ness/health/physical-activity-resources/chair-yoga.aspx

Cleveland Clinic. (2022a, April 8). *Introduction to chair yoga: a mindful, simple yet effective practice* [Video]. YouTube. https://www.youtube.com/watch?v= w4py2Gjfkqw

Cleveland Clinic. (2022b, April 8). *Introduction to chair yoga: a mindful, simple yet effective practice* [Video]. YouTube. https://www.youtube.com/watch?v= w4py2Gjfkqw

Cleveland Clinic. (2022c, April 8). *Introduction to chair yoga: a mindful, simple yet effective practice* [Video]. YouTube. https://www.youtube.com/watch?v=w4py2Gjfkqw

Cronkleton, E. (2023, June 20). *Yoga for weight loss.* Healthline. https://www.healthline.com/health/yoga-for-weight-loss

Crouch, M. (2023, October 3). *How 2 minutes of exercise can help you live longer.* AARP. https://www.aarp.org/health/healthy-living/info-2021/exercise- and-longevity.html

Davids, J. (2018, September 14). *6 reasons seniors should eat omega-3s.* Home Care Assistance - Fox Cities. https://www.homecareassistanceoshkosh.com/ omega-fatty-acids-for-seniors/

Davis, J. (2023, May 8). Live Whole Health #170: Chair yoga for the heart - VA News. *VA News.* https://news.va.gov/119507/live-whole-health-170-chair-yoga-for-the-heart/

Department of Health & Human Services. (n.d.). *Nutrition needs when you're over 65.* Better Health Channel. https://www.better-health.vic.gov.au/health/healthyliving/Nutrition-needs-when-youre-over-65

E-Ryt, P. J. (2017a, April 26). *Chair Yoga Precautions - Yoga Teacher Training blog.* Yoga Teacher Training Blog. https://www.yoga-teacher-training.org/2012/02/06/chair-yoga-precautions/

E-Ryt, P. J. (2017b, April 26). *Chair Yoga Precautions for students - Yoga Teacher Training blog.* Yoga Teacher Training Blog. https://www.yoga-teacher-training.org/2012/03/21/chair-yoga-precautions-for-students/

Exercise and aging: extending independence in older adults. (1993, May 1). PubMed. https://pubmed.ncbi.nlm.nih.gov/8486296/

Exercising more than recommended could lengthen life, study suggests. (2022, July 29). News. https://www.hsph.harvard.edu/news/hsph-in-the-news/exercising-more-than-recommended-could-lengthen-life-study-suggests/ ExpertVillage

Leaf Group. (2020, December 16). *Chair Yoga for Seniors: Mountain pose* [Video]. YouTube. https://www.youtube.com/watch?v=L6BjfH94J1A

Feller, A. (n.d.). *12 awesome Ways to Measure your Non-Scale Victories | Life by Daily Burn*. Life by Daily Burn. https://daily-burn.com/life/health/weight-loss-success-non-scale-victories/

Fiorito, R. (2017a, February 17). *De-Stress Instantly with This Easy Chair Yoga Flow*. PureWow. https://www.purewow.com/wellness/chair-yoga-poses

Fiorito, R. (2017b, February 17). *De-Stress Instantly with This Easy Chair Yoga Flow*. PureWow. https://www.purewow.com/wellness/chair-yoga-poses Fiorito, R. (2017c, February 17). *De-Stress Instantly with This Easy Chair Yoga Flow*. PureWow. https://www.purewow.com/wellness/chair-yoga-poses

Furtado, G. E., Chupel, M. U., Carvalho, H. M., Souza, N. R., Ferreira, J. P., & Teixeira, A. M. (2016). Effects of a chair-yoga exercises on stress hormone levels, daily life activities, falls and physical fitness in institutionalized older adults. *Complementary Therapies in Clinical Practice*, *24*, 123–129. https://doi.org/10.1016/j.ctcp.2016.05.012

Galantino, M. L., Green, L., DeCesari, J. A., MacKain, N. A., Rinaldi, S. M., Stevens, M., Wurst, V. R., Marsico, R., Nell, M., & Mao, J. J. (2012). Safety and feasibility of modified chair-yoga on functional outcome among elderly at risk for falls. *International Journal of Yoga*, *5*(2), 146. https://doi.org/10.4103/0973-6131.98242

GoodRX - error. (n.d.). https://www.goodrx.com/well-being/movement-exercise/chair-yoga

Haeger, C., Mümken, S., O'Sullivan, J. L., Spang, R. P., Voigt-Antons, J., Stockburger, M., Dräger, D., & Gellert, P. (2022). Mobility enhancement among older adults 75 + in rural areas: Study protocol of the MOBILE randomized controlled trial. *BMC Geriatrics*, *22*(1). https://doi.org/10.1186/ s12877-021-02739-0

Head down Chair yoga (Seated forward fold pose on chair) | Yoga sequences, benefits, variations, and Sanskrit pronunciation | Tummee.com. (2017, October 15). Tummee.com. https://www.tummee.com/yoga-poses/head-down-chair

Hellicar, L. (2022, September 16). *What is yogic breathing? Benefits and how to try it.* https://www.medicalnewstoday.com/articles/what-is-yogic-breathing

High Desert Yogi. (2021, July 20). *5 min SEATED STRETCH - quick chair yoga work break for beginners* [Video]. YouTube. https://www.youtube.com/watch?v=xRH1To_xyr8

Human Kinetics. (n.d.). *Modified chair yoga poses.* https://us.humankinetics.com/blogs/excerpt/modified-chair-yoga-poses

Isaac, B. (2023, October 19). *5 tips for promoting mobility in older adults.* Ambience In-Home Care. https://ambienceinhomecare.com/how-to-promote-mobility-in-elderly/

Jeffries, T. Y., & Jeffries, T. Y. (2023a, February 21). *13 chair yoga poses for seniors.* Yoga Journal. https://www.yogajournal.com/practice/chair-yoga-for- seniors/

Jeffries, T. Y., & Jeffries, T. Y. (2023b, February 21). *13 chair yoga poses for seniors.* Yoga Journal. https://www.yogajournal.com/practice/chair-yoga-for- seniors/

Jeffries, T. Y., & Jeffries, T. Y. (2023c, August 13). *13 Chair yoga poses anyone can do.* Yoga Journal. https://www.yogajournal.com/yoga-101/types-of-yoga/ chair-yoga-poses/

Jenny Campbell Yoga. (2019, July 14). *20 minute All-Levels chair yoga* [Video]. YouTube. https://www.youtube.com/watch?v=CMjZ2Ux4NwQ

Junková, S. (2022, August 31). Yoga for seniors + 5 breathing exercises (Pranayama) for older adults. *Prana Sutra Yoga.* https://www.prana-sutra.com/post/yoga-pranayama-for-seniors-older-adults

Kamau, C. (2023, September 1). *Chair Yoga Hip Openers: Simple Stretches For Reduced Pain & Increased Flexibility*. BetterMe Blog. https://betterme.world/articles/chair-yoga-hip-openers/

Kovacevic, L. (2023, July 13). *Seated Yoga: 16 Chair Yoga Poses For Beginners*. Wakeout | Healthy Work. https://wakeout.app/chair-yoga-poses/

LBX Fitness. (2020a, September 10). *5 minute | Seated yoga warmup or cool down* [Video]. YouTube. https://www.youtube.com/watch?v=0JMbAhoBQJQ

LBX Fitness. (2020b, September 10). *5 minute | Seated yoga warmup or cool down* [Video]. YouTube. https://www.youtube.com/watch?v=0JMbAhoBQJQ

Lcsw, M. D. (2021, September 30). *6 Benefits of exercise on Mental Health - Blue Moon Senior Counseling*. Blue Moon Senior Counseling. https://bluemoonseniorcounseling.com/6-benefits-of-exercise-on-mental-health/

LEAP Service. (2014, April 15). *Gentle Chair Yoga Routine - 25 minutes* [Video]. YouTube. https://www.youtube.com/watch?v=KEjiXtb2hRg

Lifestyle, S. (2021a, October 25). Top 10 chair yoga Positions for Seniors [Infographic]. *Senior Lifestyle*. https://www.seniorlifestyle.com/resources/ blog/infographic-top-10-chair-yoga-positions-for-seniors/

Lifestyle, S. (2021b, October 25). Top 10 chair yoga Positions for Seniors [Infographic]. *Senior Lifestyle*. https://www.seniorlifestyle.com/resources/ blog/infographic-top-10-chair-yoga-positions-for-seniors/

Lifestyle, S. (2021c, October 25). Top 10 chair yoga Positions for Seniors [Infographic]. *Senior Lifestyle*. https://www.seniorlifestyle.com/resources/ blog/infographic-top-10-chair-yoga-positions-for-seniors/

Lifestyle, S. (2021d, October 25). Top 10 chair yoga Positions for Seniors [Infographic]. *Senior Lifestyle*. https://www.seniorlifestyle.com/resources/ blog/infographic-top-10-chair-yoga-positions-for-seniors/

Lifestyle, S. (2021e, October 25). Top 10 chair yoga Positions for Seniors [Infographic]. *Senior Lifestyle*. https://www.seniorlifestyle.com/resources/ blog/info-graphic-top-10-chair-yoga-positions-for-seniors/

Lifestyle, S. (2021f, October 25). Top 10 chair yoga Positions for Seniors [Infographic]. *Senior Lifestyle*. https://www.seniorlifestyle.com/resources/ blog/info-graphic-top-10-chair-yoga-positions-for-seniors/

Lifestyle, S. (2021g, October 25). Top 10 chair yoga Positions for Seniors [Infographic]. *Senior Lifestyle*. https://www.seniorlifestyle.com/resources/ blog/info-graphic-top-10-chair-yoga-positions-for-seniors/

McGonigle, A., & McGonigle, A. (2022, November 28). *5 ways to practice half moon pose*. Yoga Journal. https://www.yogajournal.com/practice/ways-to- prac-tice-half-moon-pose/

Mighty Health. (2023, May 20). *Gentle chair yoga for joint mobility and arthritis pain* [Video]. YouTube. https://www.youtube.com/watch?v=E-5l1rTLuEI

Mph, C. a. M. (2021, December 6). *Yoga for weight loss: Benefits beyond burning calories*. Harvard Health. https://www.health.harvard.edu/blog/yoga-for-weight-loss-bene-fits-beyond-burning-calories-202112062650

Ms, M. a. a. M. (2019, March 13). *Can exercise extend your life?* Harvard Health. https://www.health.harvard.edu/blog/can-exercise-ex-tend-your-life-2019031316207

Nieves, J. W. (2003). Calcium, vitamin D, and nutrition in elderly adults. *Clinics in Geriatric Medicine, 19*(2), 321–335. https://doi.org/10.1016/s0749-0690(02)00073-3

Nutrition as We Age: Healthy Eating with the Dietary Guidelines - News & Events | health.gov. (n.d.). https://health.gov/news/202107/nutrition-we-age-healthy - eating-dietary-guidelines

Online Yoga Teaching. (2021a, May 10). *Delicious Chair Yoga | 76 min | Intermediate and Advanced Level #chairyoga #iyengaryoga* [Video]. YouTube. https://www.youtube.com/watch?v=4wyKuen2wLw

Online Yoga Teaching. (2021b, May 10). *Delicious Chair Yoga | 76 min | Intermediate and Advanced Level #chairyoga #iyengaryoga* [Video]. YouTube. https://www.youtube.com/watch?v=4wyKuen2wLw

Pagoda Yoga. (2023, February 8). *15 mins Chair yoga for strong core & weight loss || Full body results* [Video]. YouTube. https://www.youtube.com/watch?v=xxSh3QVbaDc

Paradigm Yoga. (2023, March 25). *Energizing Chair Yoga | Morning Yoga for Seniors | 20 Minute Yoga | Chair exercises* [Video]. YouTube. https://www.youtube.com/watch?v=ktx_7pc3iVc

Park, J., & McCaffrey, R. (2012). Chair Yoga: Benefits for Community-Dwelling Older Adults with Osteoarthritis. *Journal of Gerontological Nursing*, *38*(5), 12–22. https://doi.org/10.3928/00989134-20120411-50

Pohlman, D. (2020, July 29). Challenging chair yoga exercises. *Man Flow Yoga*. https://manflowyoga.com/blog/challenging-yoga-exercises-you-can-do-on-a-chair/

Rachel Scott. (2023a, February 20). *5 Awesome Chair Yoga Poses! Yoga Practice and Teaching Tips with Rachel* [Video]. YouTube. https://www.youtube.com/watch?v=LgjA6AQDN3k

Rachel Scott. (2023b, February 20). *5 Awesome Chair Yoga Poses! Yoga Practice and Teaching Tips with Rachel* [Video]. YouTube. https://www.youtube.com/watch?v=LgjA6AQDN3k

Rachel Scott. (2023c, February 20). *5 Awesome Chair Yoga Poses! Yoga Practice and Teaching Tips with Rachel* [Video]. YouTube. https://www.youtube.com/watch?v=LgjA6AQDN3k

Revolved Half Moon Pose Chair Elbow Block Yoga (Parivrtta Ardha Chandrasana Chair Elbow Block) | Yoga sequences, benefits, variations, and Sanskrit Pronunciation | Tummee.com. (2019, September 8). Tummee.com. https:// www.tumm ee.com/yoga-poses/revolved-half-moon-pose-chair-elbow- block

Ryan. (2023, July 12). *Best chair yoga poses for back pain - Start standing.* Start Standing. https://www.startstanding.org/sitting-back-pain/best-chair-yo ga- poses-for-back-pain/

Ryt, A. P. (2022a, April 22). *The history and practice of Iyengar Yoga.* Verywell Fit. https://www.verywellfit.com/why-alignment-matters-3566939

Ryt, A. P. (2022b, November 4). *10 chair yoga poses you can do at home.* Verywell Fit. https://www.verywellfit.com/chair-yoga-poses-3567189

Ryt, A. P. (2022c, November 4). *10 chair yoga poses you can do at home.* Verywell Fit. https://www.verywellfit.com/chair-yoga-poses-3567189

Ryt, A. P. (2022d, November 4). *10 chair yoga poses you can do at home.* Verywell Fit. https://www.verywellfit.com/chair-yoga-poses-3567189

Ryt, A. P. (2022e, November 4). *10 chair yoga poses you can do at home.* Verywell Fit. https://www.verywellfit.com/chair-yoga-poses-3567189

SarahBethYoga. (2022a, July 25). *20 minute CHAIR Yoga for Beginners, Seniors & Desk Workers | Full Body Stretch* [Video]. YouTube. https://www.youtube.c om/ watch?v=7yjPnhRbcV0

SarahBethYoga. (2022b, July 25). *20 minute CHAIR Yoga for Beginners, Seniors & Desk Workers | Full Body Stretch* [Video]. YouTube. https://www.youtube.c om/ watch?v=7yjPnhRbcV0

SarahBethYoga. (2022c, July 25). *20 minute CHAIR Yoga for Beginners, Seniors & Desk Workers | Full Body Stretch* [Video]. YouTube. https://www.youtube.c om/ watch?v=7yjPnhRbcV0

SarahBethYoga. (2022d, December 5). *10 minute CHAIR Yoga for Beginners, Seniors & Desk Workers | Tight Hips Stretch* [Video]. YouTube. https://www.youtube.com/watch?v=tWxKPB1uApU

SeniorShape Fitness. (2020, September 29). *Senior & Beginner Workout - 15 minute Gentle Chair Yoga* [Video]. YouTube. https://www.youtube.com/watch?v=WkYz1g47Hj0

SeniorShape Fitness. (2021a, April 19). *Chair Yoga Stretch for Beginners, Seniors & Everyone || 30 minutes* [Video]. YouTube. https://www.youtube.com/watch?v=pciXaO4wtug

SeniorShape Fitness. (2021b, April 19). *Chair Yoga Stretch for Beginners, Seniors & Everyone || 30 minutes* [Video]. YouTube. https://www.youtube.com/watch?v=pciXaO4wtug

SeniorShape Fitness. (2022a, March 14). *Chair Yoga Stretch & strength // Seated exercises for seniors & beginners* [Video]. YouTube. https://www.youtube.com/watch?v=gXB3NhOAalk

SeniorShape Fitness. (2022b, March 14). *Chair Yoga Stretch & strength // Seated exercises for seniors & beginners* [Video]. YouTube. https://www.youtube.com/watch?v=gXB3NhOAalk

Sites, S. (2023, August 16). *A Senior's Guide To Chair Yoga*. Discovery Village. https://www.discoveryvillages.com/senior-living-blog/a-seniors-guide-to- chair-yoga/

Smith, E. N. (2023, March 2). *Which muscles are you using in your yoga practice? A new study provides the answers*. YogaUOnline. https://yogauonline.com/yoga- practice-teaching-tips/yoga-anatomy/which-muscles-are-you-using-in- your-yoga-practice-a-new-study-provides-the-answers/

Target Yoga. (2021, March 4). *YOGA FOR SENIORS WITH BAD KNEES - Chair Yoga For Seniors With Knee Pain* [Video]. YouTube. https://www.youtube. com/watch?v=S73wD0AMTmQ

The National Council on Aging. (n.d.). https://www.ncoa.org/article/how-to-stay- hydrated-for-better-health

The Sunflower Channel. (2019, August 10). *Chair Yoga: Gentle Warm Up & Short Routine* [Video]. YouTube. https://www.youtube.com/watch ? v=AjpDXLTlb7A

Training, T. A. (2023, October 3). Chair Yoga For Seniors: The Ultimate Guide To A Healthy And Active Lifestyle. *Type A Training.* https://www.typeatra in ing.com/blog/chair-yoga-for-seniors-the-ultimate-guide-to-a-healthy-and- active-lifestyle/

Trinh, E. (2019, June 28). 5 Accurate ways to measure progress without a scale. *Aaptiv.* https://aaptiv.com/magazine/measuring-progress-beyo nd-scale/ UHBlog. (2020, March 13). How chair yoga can expand your practice. *University Hospitals.* https://www.uhhospitals.org/blog/articles/2020/03/how-chair-yoga-can-expand-your-practice
Vallath, N. (2010). Perspectives on *Yoga* inputs in the management of chronic pain. *Indian Journal of Palliative Care*, *16*(1), 1. https://doi.org/10.4103/0973-1075.63127

Vitamin D and calcium. (n.d.). Johns Hopkins Medicine. https://www.hopkinsmedicine.org/health/wellness-and-prevention/vitamin-d-and-calcium

Vive Health. (2020, February 5). *Seated forward bend chair stretch* [Video]. YouTube.https://www.youtube.com/watch?v=QRIKGOUJILs

WebMD Editorial Contributors. (2021, March 24). *What to know about fish oil dosage for older adults*. WebMD. https://www.webmd.com/healthy-aging/what-to-know-about-fish-oil-dosage-for-older-adults

YMCANorth. (2020, April 28). *Chair yoga practice for seniors! (20-Minute routine)* [Video]. YouTube. https://www.youtube.com/watch?v=2IuWm9wKqAk

Yoga With Adriene. (2017a, July 23). *Chair Yoga - Yoga For Seniors | Yoga With Adriene* [Video]. YouTube. https://www.youtube.com/watch?v=-Ts01MC2mIo

Yoga With Adriene. (2017b, July 23). *Chair Yoga - Yoga For Seniors | Yoga With Adriene* [Video]. YouTube. https://www.youtube.com/watch?v=-Ts01MC2mIo

Yoga with Kassandra. (2019a, July 11). *Gentle chair yoga for beginners and seniors* [Video]. YouTube. https://www.youtube.com/watch?v=1DYH5ud3zHo

Yoga with Kassandra. (2019b, July 11). *Gentle chair yoga for beginners and seniors* [Video]. YouTube. https://www.youtube.com/watch?v=1DYH5ud3zHo

Yoga with Kassandra. (2019c, July 11). *Gentle chair yoga for beginners and seniors*

[Video]. YouTube. https://www.youtube.com/watch?v=1DYH5ud3zHo
Yoga with Kassandra. (2023, September 4). *15 min Chair Yoga Class for Seniors & Beginners* [Video]. YouTube. https://www.youtube.com/watch?v=P0Yos-Dn-ExM

Yoga15abi. (2022, September 16). *Yoga For Balance, Body Control And Coordination - Yoga 15*. Yoga 15. https://yoga15.com/article/yoga-for-balance-body-control-and-coordination/

Your first chair yoga class in a senior center. (n.d.). https://www.streetdirectory. com/travel_guide/24349/yoga/your_first_chair_yoga_class_in_a_senior_center.html

ZindzyGracia. (2023, November 15). *20 Chair Yoga Exercises That'll Take You From Couch Potato To Future Yogi*. BetterMe Blog. https://betterme.world/articles/chair-yoga-exercises/

Zolotow, N. (2023, February 8). *Chair Yoga: A Guide to Resources*. Yoga for Times of Change. https://www.yogafortimesofchange.com/chair-yoga-a-guide-to-resources/

Quick and Effective Wall Pilates for Seniors

50+ Easy Step-by-Step Poses, to Improve Balance, Alleviate Pain, Strengthen the Core, to Enhance Flexibility & Posture in Under 10 Minutes a Day.

Laurel Harris

INTRODUCTION

RECLAIM YOUR VITALITY, REDEFINE YOUR GOLDEN YEARS WITH WALL PILATES

Waking up with the sun, not the sting of stiffness in your lower back, sounds great, right? A gentle stretch, a sip of coffee, and you're ready to greet the day – not with a wince, but with a smile. Your grandkids erupt in giggles as you chase them through the sun-dappled park, your knees bending with ease. You join your friends for a lively dinner, your laugh echoing through the room, fuelled by newfound energy and confidence. This isn't a fantasy; it's the life waiting for you on the other side of this book, your guide to reclaiming your golden years and rediscovering the vibrant potential that lies within.

But it wasn't always like this. We've all lived the creeping tide of aches and pains that come with the years. The groan as you rise from a chair, the sharp pang in your shoulder when reaching for a high shelf, the constant reminder that your body isn't the same as it used to be. Maybe you've tried it all – expensive creams, endless stretches, even that questionable yoga pose that left you feeling more bruised than balanced. And yet, the nagging limitations remained, casting a shadow over your days.

The truth? You don't have to settle for this. You don't have to let age dictate your activity level, social life, or joy. Wall Pilates is a secret weapon waiting for you right in your own home, requiring no fancy equipment or gruelling workouts.

Forget the intimidating gym memberships; Wall Pilates is your gentle, low-impact solution to pain relief, increased mobility, and a renewed zest for life – all in just 10 minutes a day. It's designed for seniors like you, understanding your aches, limitations, and deepest desires. Imagine:

Say goodbye to daily aches and pains: Wall Pilates' targeted movements gently stretch and strengthen your muscles, reducing inflammation and improving flexibility. No more wincing as you bend, no more stiffness holding you back.

Moving with newfound confidence: Forget the fear of falls and the frustration of limited mobility. Wall Pilates builds core strength and improves balance, giving you the freedom to move with ease and grace, whether it's dancing with your grandkids or navigating a bustling market.

Boosting your energy levels: No more feeling sluggish and drained. Wall Pilates' controlled movements and mindful breathing techniques increase circulation and oxygen flow, leaving you energised and ready to tackle the day with a smile.

Rekindling your social life: Reclaim your independence and reconnect with your loved ones. As your mobility and confidence improve, so does your social circle. You'll be the life of the party, sharing stories and laughter with newfound enthusiasm.

Feeling empowered and in control: Ditch the dependence on painkillers and take charge of your well-being. Wall Pilates is your self-directed path to a healthier, happier you, leaving you proud and in control of your health.

But don't just take my word for it. This book contains exercises to relieve pain and rediscover your youthful energy through Wall Pilates. Transformative power is waiting for you on the pages ahead.

And I'm not just any author. For years, I grappled with the same aches and limitations as you. Acupuncture, endless stretches; from trendy fads to costly programs – I tried it all, searching for relief that didn't involve surgery or harsh medications while hoping to outrun the ache in my knees, the groan in my shoulders. Then I discovered Wall Pilates, and it changed everything. The pain lessened, my energy increased, and my zest for life returned. Now, I'm here to share this life-changing secret with you, the secret that helped me reclaim my golden years and write this book with a heart full of hope and a smile on my face.

This book is your roadmap to a better you. Inside, you'll find:

Over 50 easy-to-follow Wall Pilates poses: No complicated sequences or intimidating jargon. Start today with clear, step-by-step instructions with modifications for different fitness levels, ensuring you find the perfect routine for your needs.

Beautiful illustrations: Visualise each pose with clear, detailed illustrations that guide you through every movement, ensuring you perform each exercise safely and effectively.

Targeted routines: Choose from routines designed to address specific concerns, whether improving balance, reducing back pain, or boosting flexibility.

Expert tips and safety advice: Get the most out of your workouts with helpful tips on form, breathing, and preventing injuries.

Every morning promises a fresh start, a canvas to paint with vibrant experiences. But for those of us in our golden years, that canvas can sometimes feel faded, dulled by the aches and limitations that whisper with age. We yearn for the days when movement felt effortless, laughter flowed freely, and life brimmed with possibility.

Some might see age as a finish line, a slowing down, a quiet surrender to aches and limitations. But not us. We, the vibrant souls in our golden years, know better. We've climbed mountains, chased dreams, and embraced every twist and turn life threw. Now, it's time to redefine what "aging" means. As Jeff Bridges eloquently says, "Being healthy is one of the greatest gifts." It's a gift to ourselves, granting independence, energy, and the ability to keep chasing those sunsets with the people we love. And it's a gift to them, ensuring we're present, engaged, and ready to share adventures for years.

And like Helen Mirren said, "Keep taking chances and growing," don't retreat into self-preservation. Wall Pilates isn't about slowing down; it's about igniting a newfound spark, a gentle revolution that whispers, "This is just the beginning."

This book isn't just another promise; it's a brush dipped in hope, ready to recolour your canvas with vibrant strokes of rediscovered joy. It's your invitation to reclaim your golden years, shed your limitations, and step into a life where pain fades, energy soars and movement becomes a celebration.

Turning the page is the first step on this journey. Within these chapters, you'll find the secrets of Wall Pilates, a gentle, low-impact program designed specifically for seniors like you. It's your key to unlocking a treasure trove of benefits.

So why wait? Jump in, and let's rewrite your senior years together.

CHAPTER 1

WALL PILATES THAT CHANGE LIVES

"Embrace the change, and watch your strength unfold."

Do you sometimes gaze at pictures from your younger self, filled with a bitter-sweet mix of longing and acceptance? The body that moved with effortless grace, the spirit that embraced every adventure without hesitation – those echoes can still resonate, even if time has whispered its story on your joints. But what if you could rediscover a spark of that youthful potential, a gentle revolution nestled within the comfort of your own home?

The Evolution of Pilates for Seniors: Finding Grace in a New Chapter

The longing glance at youthful photos and the bittersweet acceptance of changes brought by time are experiences many seniors share. But just as time sculpted its story on your joints, a different force can bring about a new chapter: **Wall Pilates.**

Developed as an adaptation of the famed Joseph Pilates method, Wall Pilates reimagines movement for aging adults. With no intimidating gym equipment, no complex sequences, just your sturdy wall and a gentle exploration of your own body, it's an evolution tailor-made for the senior experience, a whisper of youthful potential rekindled in the comfort of your home.

But how did this revolution in movement come to be? The original Pilates method, emphasising core strength and flexibility, held immense promise for seniors. However, the traditional exercises often required equipment and advanced manoeuvres, posing challenges for older adults with decreased mobility or balance issues. Recognising this need, forward-thinking instructors began adapting the principles to a simpler, more accessible format called Wall Pilates: a gentle symphony of movement conducted with your trusty wall as your partner.

This adaptation isn't merely a watered-down version; it's a reinvention. By utilising the wall for support and balance, Wall Pilates allows seniors to perform exercises that might otherwise be difficult or impossible on the mat. It empowers them to rediscover the joy of movement without fearing falls or strain. It's a conversation with your body that whispers possibilities rather than limitations.

Benefits of Wall Pilates for Aging Adults

The benefits of Wall Pilates extend far beyond physical gains. It's a holistic approach to well-being, working its way into the fabric of your life, one gentle movement at a time. Here are just a few changes you can discover:

Enhanced Mobility and Flexibility: Wall Pilates stretches and strengthens vital muscle groups, improving your range of motion and reducing stiffness – a welcome antidote to the aches and limitations that can accompany aging. Imagine bending down to tie your shoes without a groan or reaching for a high shelf with newfound ease.

Improved Balance and Stability: Fear of falls can be a significant concern for seniors. Wall Pilates can help build core strength and proprioception, reducing your risk of falls and enhancing your balance. This newfound confidence allows you to navigate your world more independently and joyfully.

Reduced Pain and Discomfort: Wall Pilates' focus on gentle, low-impact movements can ease chronic pain and discomfort, particularly in the back and joints. It can even help manage conditions like arthritis by promoting flexibility and strengthening surrounding muscles.

Sharper Focus and Cognitive Function: Studies have shown that regular physical activity, like Wall Pilates, can enhance cognitive function and memory. This gentle workout can help keep your mind sharp and focused, allowing you to embrace life's challenges with a clear and present mind.

Improved Mood and Well-being: Wall Pilates's rhythmic movements and mindful focus can provide a powerful sense of calm, reducing anxiety and stress. This newfound emotional balance can spill over into all aspects of your life, fostering a sense of well-being and happiness.

Wall Pilates isn't about chasing a lost ideal of youth but embracing the present with grace and acceptance. It's about rediscovering the joy of movement, the strength within, and the beauty of aging with every gentle breath and mindful flow.

Understanding the Mind-Body Connection

Wall Pilates isn't simply a collection of exercises; it's a conversation between your mind and body. Every controlled movement, every mindful breath, becomes a gentle promise of wholeness. Joseph Pilates, the creator of this system, believed that strengthening the core isn't just about physical muscles; it's about building a centre of power within, a foundation for both physical and mental well-being.

Think of it like cultivating a beautiful garden. You wouldn't just focus on tending the flowers; you'd nourish the soil, nurture the roots, and ensure a delicate balance between sunlight and water. Wall Pilates takes this approach, addressing your physical needs while tending to the fertile ground of your mind. The gentle movements cultivate a sense of calm and focus, reducing stress and anxieties that can cloud your days.

Importance of Physical Activity for Seniors

Physical activity isn't just about defying age; it's about embracing life to the fullest. As we journey through the years, our bodies might show changes, but movement offers a powerful counterpoint. Studies have shown that regular physical activity, like Wall Pilates, can not only enhance strength and flexibility but also bring a multitude of benefits:

Reduced risk of chronic diseases: Regular exercise can be a robust preventative measure against everything from heart disease and osteoporosis to diabetes and even some cancers.

Improved cognitive function: Movement keeps the mind sharp, boosting memory, focus, and overall cognitive health, helping you stay engaged and vibrant.

Enhanced mood and well-being: Physical activity releases endorphins, nature's mood elevators, combating stress and anxiety while promoting a sense of calm and well-being.

Increased independence and confidence: As your strength and balance improve, you gain the confidence to navigate your world with autonomy, reducing falls and enhancing your daily routines.

Stronger social connections: Engaging in physical activity, whether in a group setting or the comfort of your own home, can open doors to social interaction and foster a sense of community.

Keep in mind that even small steps matter. Regular Wall Pilates practice, just 10 minutes a day, can be the gentle nudge your body needs to reap the incredible rewards of movement.

How Wall Pilates Differs from Traditional Pilates

Traditional Pilates can be intimidating for seniors with its reformer machines and challenging sequences. This is where Wall Pilates steps in. Here are some key differences:

Accessibility: Wall Pilates requires no expensive equipment, just you and a sturdy wall. This makes it an ideal option for seniors who prefer to exercise in the comfort and affordability of their own homes.

Gentleness: Traditional Pilates can be rigorous, emphasising advanced exercises. Wall Pilates focuses on low-impact movements that suit different fitness levels and limitations. This allows seniors to build strength and flexibility without undue strain gradually.

Focus on balance: Wall Pilates utilises the wall as a supportive partner, enhancing balance and stability. This is especially beneficial for seniors who might be concerned about falls or have impaired balance.

Mindful movement: Unlike the high-intensity routines of some fitness programs, Wall Pilates emphasises controlled movements and mindful breathing. This focus on the present moment creates a sense of calm and promotes stress reduction.

Customisation: Wall Pilates provides extensive exercises that are customisable to individual needs and preferences. Whether your goal is to enhance flexibility, increase strength, or engage in gentle movement, a tailored Wall Pilates routine awaits you.

Think of Wall Pilates as the bridge between your youthful vitality and the wisdom of your years. It allows you to embrace the aging journey with grace and acceptance, rediscovering the joy of movement and the strength within, one gentle breath and mindful flow at a time.

Conquering Myths: Embracing Exercise As Seniors

The path to staying active as seniors and beyond can be paved with well-meaning but often misleading advice. Let's dispel some common myths and empower you to claim your movement potential confidently!

Myth 1: *"I'm too old to start exercising now."* Physical activity can always benefit you. Your body is a resilient wonder, and even small doses of movement can make a big difference. Wall Pilates's gentle nature is perfectly tailored for beginners of all ages, including seniors. Think of it as a conversation with your body, a gradual reawakening of its potential, not a race against time.

Myth 2: *"Exercise will make my aches and pains worse."* The opposite is often true! Gentle, low-impact exercises like Wall Pilates can reduce pain and discomfort. Especially in the joints, thereby promoting flexibility and strengthening surrounding muscles.

Myth 3: *"I need fancy equipment and a gym membership."* Wall Pilates requires nothing more than your determination and, you guessed it, a wall! No expensive equipment or intimidating gyms are needed. This makes it accessible and convenient for everyone, allowing you to reclaim your fitness in the comfort and privacy of your own home.

Myth 4: *"Exercise is boring and strenuous."* Wall Pilates is anything but! Its mindful movements focus on breathing, and gentle flow can be surprisingly meditative. You'll find yourself connecting with your body in a new way.

Myth 5: *"I won't see any results."* Consistency is critical, and even small changes add up. With regular Wall Pilates practice, you'll notice increased flexibility, improved balance, and a boost in energy levels. You may even find your aches and pains fading, replaced by a newfound sense of well-being and confidence.

Why Choose Wall Pilates?

So, with all the fancy exercise options, why choose Wall Pilates? Well, think of it as the gentle revolution that says, "Less is more." Here's why it might be the perfect fit for you:

Benefits on a Budget: Remember those benefits we talked about? Enhanced mobility, reduced pain, boosted energy – you get all that without breaking the bank. No fancy equipment, just you and your friendly wall.

No Gym Jitters: Forget the intimidating atmosphere of crowded gyms. Wall Pilates is your home sanctuary, where you can move at your own pace, in your pyjamas, if you desire. Cozy comfort meets effective exercise – what's not to love?

Effortless Efficiency: Wall Pilates isn't about pushing yourself to the limit. It's about intelligent movement, using your body weight and the wall's support to achieve maximum results with minimal effort. So, say goodbye to grunting and hello to graceful, mindful movement.

It's simple. Wall Pilates offers a gentle, effective way to rediscover your strength, all in the comfort of your own home. There is no pressure, just pure, unadulterated well-being waiting to be unlocked.

What you will need to start

So, are you ready to dive into the world of Wall Pilates? That's fantastic! This gentle yet powerful practice requires minimal equipment and can be done in the comfort of your own home. Here's a quick checklist to get you started:

Essentials:

Comfortable clothes: Think stretchy and sweat-wicking, allowing for freedom of movement.

Non-slip socks or bare feet: Your feet connect to the wall, so a good grip is crucial.

Spacious area: Find a clear patch of wall with enough room to move your arms and legs freely.

Optional props: A yoga mat for cushioning and a small blanket or towel for support are excellent additions.

Safety First:

Listen to your body: Don't push yourself beyond your limits. If something feels uncomfortable, stop and adjust the movement.

Mind your medical history: If you have any pre-existing conditions, consult your doctor before starting any new exercise program.

Start slow and steady: Begin with short, gentle routines and gradually increase intensity as your body adapts.

Charting Your Course:

Set realistic goals: What do you hope to achieve with Wall Pilates? Increased flexibility, better balance, or simply a fun way to move? Defining your goals helps tailor your practice.

Embrace the journey: Wall Pilates is a lifelong adventure, not a sprint. Celebrate small victories, enjoy the process, and witness the magic unfold with every mindful breath and gentle movement.

So, take a deep breath, find your wall, and embark on your Wall Pilates journey with a smile!

Monitoring Progress and Adjusting Goals

As you journey through your Wall Pilates practice, don't get hung up on the finish line. Listen to your body, respect its pace, and adjust your goals accordingly. Every bend, stretch and confident step is a triumph to savour.

Here are some tips to help you track your progress and make adjustments as needed:

Keep a simple progress log: Note how you feel before and after each session, focusing on energy levels, mood, and any specific improvements you notice.

Focus on body awareness: Pay attention to your body's signals during exercises. If something feels uncomfortable, modify the movement or take a break.

Embrace modifications: Don't be afraid to adjust exercises to suit your abilities. Wall Pilates is about gentle progress, not pushing yourself to the point of pain.

Listen to your inner cheerleader: Celebrate your achievements, no matter how small!

Your Wall Pilates journey is unique, so don't get caught up in comparing yourself to others. Trust your instincts, listen to your body, and enjoy rediscovering your strength and grace.

Recognising and Respecting Individual Limits: Your Body, Your Pace

While Wall Pilates is gentle and adaptable, honouring your body's limitations is crucial. Everybody has their own story of aches, pains, and past experiences. Some things to keep in mind:

Start slow and listen to your body: Don't jump into advanced exercises before you're ready. Begin with beginner-friendly routines and gradually increase intensity as you gain confidence.

Modifications are your friends: Remember, there's no shame in modifying exercises to suit your needs. Use props or chairs, or adapt the movements to match your comfort level.

Pain is a red flag: Stop immediately if you experience any pain during exercise. Listen to your body's warning signs and take a break or modify the movement.

Respecting your limits isn't about giving up; it's about setting yourself up for sustainable success. Listening to your body and adjusting as needed ensures a safe and enjoyable journey toward a stronger, healthier you.

***

A Sneak Peek at Your Journey: A Glimpse into the Exercise List

B EFORE WE DIVE INTO the world of specific Wall Pilates exercises, let's get you excited about the possibilities! Here's a quick taste of what awaits you:

Warm-up sequences: Gentle stretches and movements to prepare your body for safe and effective exercise.

Beginner-friendly routines: Easy-to-follow exercises focusing on core strength, balance, and flexibility.

Intermediate to Advanced challenges: As you gain confidence, the exercises will gradually increase in intensity, keeping you engaged and motivated.

Cool-down rituals: Relieve post-workout tension and promote relaxation with mindful movements and deep breathing.

This is just a sneak peek. Each exercise is carefully chosen and explained, and modifications are made to meet your needs.

Exercise List

Beginner

Warm Up: two minutes of gentle movement to get your blood flowing and joints lubricated:

Raise your arms sideways and above your head, and hold for 30 seconds.

Roll your shoulders backwards and forwards for 30 seconds.

Circle your wrists clockwise and counterclockwise for 30 seconds.

Gently bend forward, sliding your hand gently down the front of your legs, and hold for 30 seconds

Wall Roll Down:

Stand tall with your back against the wall, feet shoulder-width apart. Inhale, reach your arms overhead, lengthening your spine.

Exhale, slowly peel your spine off the wall, one vertebra at a time, starting at your head and rolling down until your back is rounded. Inhale, slowly roll your spine back up, pressing each vertebra into the wall. Repeat 5-10 times.

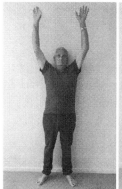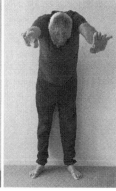

Wall Squats:

Stand back against the wall, feet hip-width apart, heel flat on the floor. Lean back slightly and slide down the wall until your thighs are parallel to the floor (or as low as comfortable).

Engage your core and keep your back straight. Press your heels into the floor and push yourself back to standing. Repeat 10-15 times.

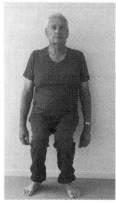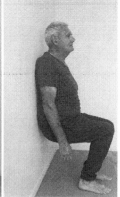

Wall Arm Circles:

Stand facing the wall, arms out to the sides at shoulder height, palms facing forward. Make small circles with your arms, increasing the size gradually as you warm up. Do ten circles forward and ten circles backward.

Cool Down: 2 minutes of deep breathing and relaxation

Stand with your back against the wall, breathe deeply and relax your muscles. Keep your breathing in check and practice a breathing exercise (*refer to Chapter four for breathing techniques*) while you clear your mind and focus on mental and physical harmony.

Final Relaxation:

Body Scan - While you relax with some meditation or a brief walk, take a moment to check in with your body and make sure it's healthy. Is the workout causing any new types of muscle or joint pain? On the other hand, have you noticed any improvement in the symptoms of any aches and pains you were experiencing before?

Make it a habit to check in with your body in this way before and after each workout. You might be misaligning yourself, practising a pose incorrectly, or there could be an unidentified problem in that area if you experience new pain.

When exercising, be careful not to strain joints or muscles that hurt before you start.

Intermediate

Warm Up: Same as Beginner

Wall Spine Stretch:

Sit on the floor with your back against the wall and your legs extended. Lean back until your back is flat against the wall and your legs are perpendicular to the floor.

Reach your arms overhead, interlace your fingers, and gently press your palms towards the ceiling. Hold for 10-30 seconds, keeping your core engaged and back flat. Do this five times, extending the seconds as comfortably as you feel.

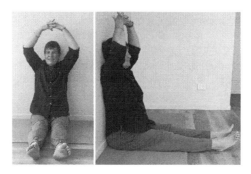

Wall Calf Stretch:

Stand facing the wall with one foot a step forward, with both heels flat on the floor. Lean and bend your front knee slightly forward so your knee is touching the wall. You should feel a stretch in your calf and Achilles tendon.

Hold for 10-30 seconds and repeat on the other side. Do this five times.

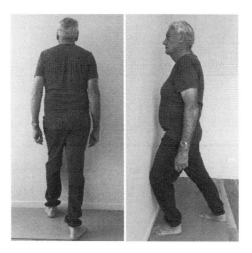

Wall Chest Opener:

Stand facing the wall with your arms bent at shoulder height, elbows aligned with your shoulders and forearms against the wall.

Slowly open your chest by pressing your arms against the wall and gently arching your back. Hold for 10-30 seconds. Do this three times.

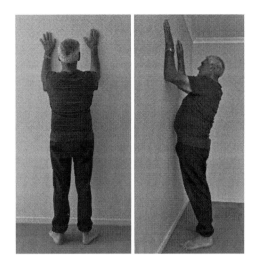

Wall Leg Lifts:

Lay on your back, bending your legs with your feet resting flat on the floor. Press your lower back into the mat and lift one leg straight towards the ceiling, keeping your core engaged.

Gradually lower the leg onto the mat and repeat the movement with the other leg. Do 10-15 lifts per leg.

Cool Down: Same as Beginner

Advanced

Warm Up: Same as Beginner

Wall Plank:

Stand facing the wall, arms bent at shoulder height, elbows aligned with your shoulders, and forearms against the wall. Activate your core muscles and keep your body straight from your head to your heels.

Hold for 30 seconds to one minute, or as long as possible.

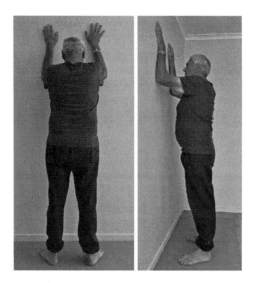

Wall Hamstring Stretch:

Lay on the floor with the wall in front of you, with one leg extended straight up the wall and the other foot flat on the floor with your knee bent. Lean forward towards your straight leg and reach towards your toes; you should feel a stretch in your hamstring.

Hold for 10-30 seconds and repeat on the other side. Do this five times.

Wall Shoulder Bridge:

Lay on your back, bending your legs and resting your feet flat on the floor. Press your heels into the floor and lift your hips off the mat, squeezing your glutes and keeping your back flat.

Hold for 10-30 seconds and slowly lower back down. Repeat five times.

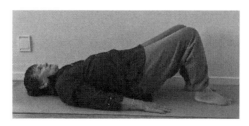

Cool Down: Same as Beginner

So, gaze at that picture of your younger self as you get to exercise, and I will see you in the next chapter, where we talk about *flexibility*.

CHAPTER 2

IMPORTANCE OF IMPROVED FLEXIBILITY

"Flexibility, the key to resilience. Bend, but never break."

Have you ever felt that ache in your back after reaching for a mug? Or the frustrating struggle to tie your shoes without grimacing? Well, if you have, you're not alone. What would the opposite feel like? Reaching for a high shelf without a groan, bending down to touch your toes with a smile, and twisting your body with newfound grace. Improved flexibility is about rediscovering the freedom of movement and embracing the vibrant possibilities that come with a supple body and a youthful spirit.

The Role Of Flexibility In Aging Gracefully

Why is flexibility so crucial, especially as we age gracefully? It is true that our bodies naturally experience a decline in flexibility as we age. Collagen production slows down, muscle fibres shorten, and joint cartilage thins. But this isn't a story of inevitable decline! Studies from the Mayo Clinic and Harvard University show that regular flexibility training can significantly improve your range of motion, even at an advanced age.

Understanding Age-Related Changes in Flexibility

The good news is that our potential for improved flexibility resides just like a dusty attic holding forgotten treasures. While age brings changes, it doesn't have to dictate limitations. Understanding how these changes manifest can empower us to navigate them with gentle movements and mindful awareness.

Muscle loss: Muscle mass naturally declines with age, impacting our strength and flexibility.

Joint changes: Cartilage wear and tear can decrease joint mobility and stiffness.

Reduced proprioception: Our body's awareness of its position in space can diminish, leading to an increased risk of falls.

Despite these changes, the human body holds an incredible capacity for adaptation. Regular stretching and targeted exercises can help us regain lost ground, increase our range of motion, and unlock a vibrant list of benefits.

Benefits of Increased Range of Motion for Seniors

Improved flexibility isn't just about touching your toes (although that's pretty cool too!) It's about reclaiming the freedom to move confidently and efficiently, paving the way for a healthier and happier you. Here are just a few things you can discover:

Reduced discomfort: Gentle stretching can ease pain and remove unnecessary discomfort when doing things, particularly in the back and joints, thereby improving overall comfort and well-being.

Increased stability: Increased range of motion strengthens core muscles and improves proprioception, reducing the risk of falls and promoting graceful movement.

Boosted energy levels: Regular stretching can improve circulation and increase oxygen flow, energising and revitalising you.

Stress reduction: The gentle movements and mindful focus of stretching can lower stress hormones and promote relaxation, leaving you feeling calmer and more optimistic.

Better confidence: With improved flexibility, everyday tasks become more accessible and enjoyable, fostering independence and self-reliance.

The journey towards increased flexibility is not a race but a gentle dance with your body.

Incorporating Stretching into Daily Life: Making it a Gentle Habit.

The beauty of improved flexibility is that it doesn't require expensive equipment or strenuous workouts. You can easily incorporate gentle stretching into your daily routine, making it a sustainable habit for a lifetime:

Start small and listen to your body: Don't push yourself beyond your comfort zone. Begin with short, five-minute stretches before or after your usual activities.

Focus on mindful movement: Pay attention to your breath and sensations during each stretch. Breathe deeply and move slowly, savouring the release of tension.

Target all major muscle groups: Don't neglect any area. Include neck, shoulders, back, hips, legs, and finger stretches!

Find your flexibility flow: Discover activities you enjoy, like yoga, Pilates (especially Wall Pilates!), or even tai chi.

Addressing Common Myths About Flexibility

Flexibility is a word often cloaked in misconceptions. Some believe it's reserved for gymnasts and contortionists, while others fear it's synonymous with painful contortions. But cast those fears aside. Improved flexibility is not about contorting your body into a pretzel; it's about befriending your muscles, whispering sweet, and rediscovering the joy of flowing freely through life.

Myth 1: *"You're 'too old' to be flexible."* That's not true. Flexibility is a lifelong adventure. You can learn a new language at any age, bake a delicious cake at any stage in life, or cultivate supple muscles at any age.

Myth 2: *"I'm not a gymnast."* Who says flexibility is for the gymnasts alone? You don't need to do all the extra things like putting both your legs around your neck (although if you want that, I bet you can get that!); you need to bend and pick things without hearing a snap.

Myth 3: *"Stretching hurts, so it must be bad."* While a slight twinge is usual, a sharp pain is a red flag. Listen to your body and modify exercises if needed. Ensuring a safe and pain-free path toward an increased range of motion is part of the journey.

Tailoring Your Wall Pilates Journey to Your Unique Flexibility Needs

The beauty of Wall Pilates lies in its versatility. Whether you aim to reduce pain, improve balance, or move more efficiently, you can tailor your practice accordingly. Focus on exercises that target specific areas, adjust their intensity to match your needs, and create a unique choreography of movement that reflects your personal goals.

Beginner? Start with gentle stretches, focusing on core strengthening and basic movements. Wall Pilates offers beginner-friendly routines that build a solid foundation for progress.

Intermediate and Advanced? Push yourself with advanced exercises that expand your range of motion and focus on particular muscle groups.

Limited mobility? Don't despair! Use props, adjust postures, and listen to your body's whispers to find your perfect flow.

Progress takes time and patience. Your flexibility journey is a personal dance, not a race to the finish line.

Cooling Down for Enhanced Flexibility

After your flexibility workout, remember to cool down! This helps to:

Prevent muscle soreness: Gentle stretches and slow movements cool down your muscles and prevent post-workout discomfort.

Promote relaxation: Deep breathing and mindful movements help you transition from movement to stillness, leaving you feeling refreshed and rejuvenated.

Maintain flexibility gains: Regular cool-down routines help your muscles retain the increased range of motion you achieved during your workout.

Flexibility Challenges and Solutions: Every Journey Has Its Twists and Turns

Even the smoothest waltz has its moments of unexpected steps. Keep going even if you encounter challenges on your flexibility journey.

Here are some solutions:

Pain? Stop the exercise promptly and seek advice from a healthcare professional if necessary. Remember, discomfort is not a sign of achievement in flexibility training.

Plateaus? Don't be afraid to challenge yourself with new exercises or modifications.

Flexibility Assessment for Seniors

Gentle Touch Test: Reach for your toes without bending your knees. How far do your fingers reach? This gives a basic sense of hamstring and calf flexibility.

Sit and Reach Test: Sit on the floor with legs straight and reach forward. Can you touch your toes or feel tightness in your hamstrings and lower back?

Shoulder Rotation Test: Raise your arms to the sides and make small circles. Do your shoulders move smoothly, or do you feel stiffness?

These are just simple starting points; write down your results so you can compare them later. Remember to listen to your body and do not push yourself beyond your comfort zone.

Flexibility Maintenance Between Sessions

Short, mindful stretches throughout the day: Take a few minutes to gently stretch your neck, shoulders, and back while standing in line at the grocery store or during your morning coffee break.

Active movements: Incorporate simple movements like arm circles and leg swings into your daily routine.

Focus on hydration: Water is crucial for keeping your muscles and joints lubricated, which enhances flexibility. Aim for eight glasses of water per day.

Adapting Flexibility Exercises to Personal Goals

Identify your goals: To improve your posture, reduce pain, or feel more limber. Tailor your exercises accordingly.

Choose exercises that target specific areas: If you have tight hamstrings, focus on stretches for your lower body. If you have tight shoulders, prioritise upper back and arm exercises.

Listen to your body and modify as needed: Don't be afraid to modify exercises to make them comfortable and safe. Remember, progress is personal.

Flexibility Exercises for Specific Joints

Neck: Gentle head rolls and chin tucks can help improve neck flexibility and reduce stiffness.

Shoulders: Arm circles, shoulder shrugs, and gentle chest openers can improve shoulder mobility and reduce pain.

Spine: Cat-cow poses and gentle twists can help improve spinal flexibility and posture.

Hips and knees: Hip circles and leg swings can improve hip and knee flexibility and reduce stiffness.

Enhancing Flexibility for Better Posture

Focus on stretches for your chest, shoulders, and back: These muscles often become tight, leading to poor posture.

Strengthen your core muscles: A strong core supports your spine, improving posture and flexibility.

Practice mindful movement throughout your day: Be aware of your posture and gently correct yourself when needed.

Flexibility for Improved Circulation and Joint Health

Regular stretching improves blood flow to your joints, keeping them lubricated and healthy. Even minor improvements in flexibility can significantly impact your overall health and well-being.

***

Preview of Exercise List in This Chapter

GET READY TO EMBARK on your flexibility journey! The exercises below provide gentle stretches tailored for seniors, targeting specific muscle groups and joints. We'll also explore advanced exercises for those who want to push their limits, always emphasising safety and mindful movement.

This is just a glimpse of the exciting world of flexibility waiting for you. Be prepared to rediscover the joy of movement, the freedom of a supple body, and the vibrant possibilities that unfold with each gentle stretch.

Exercise List

Beginner:

Warm-up (two minutes):

Gentle Neck Rolls: Slowly roll your head in a circular motion, forward and backward. Do this for one minute

Perform Arm Circles: Rotate your arms in small circles (letting your hands go slightly above your head), forward and backward, 30 seconds. Focus on shoulder mobility.

Ankle Pumps: Point and flex your ankles down and up. Feel the stretch in your calves. Do this for 30 seconds.

Wall Hip Flexor Stretch (One minute):

Position yourself in front of the wall with your feet spaced hip-width apart. Lean back and place hands shoulder-height on the wall for support.

Lift one leg slightly and gently pull your knee towards your chest, feeling a stretch in the front of your thigh. Hold for 30 seconds each leg.

Wall Shoulder Stretch (One minute):

Position yourself in front of the wall with your feet spaced hip-width apart. Reach both arms overhead, fingers interlaced. Lean your body against the wall, gently pressing your palms.

Feel a stretch in your shoulders and chest. Hold for 30 seconds, then repeat.

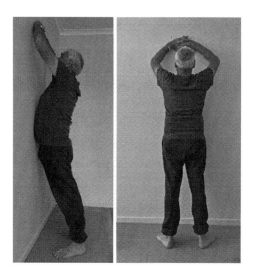

Wall Cat-Cow Stretch (10 repetitions):

Start on all fours, knees hip-width apart and hands shoulder-width apart. On an inhale, arch your back and bring your chin towards your chest (cow pose). When exhaling, lower your back and raise your head. (cat pose). Breathe smoothly and repeat ten times.

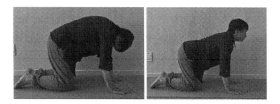

Wall Side Stretch (30 seconds on each side):

Position yourself in front of the wall with your feet spaced hip-width apart. Reach one arm overhead as high as possible and place your hand on the wall above your head; you should feel a stretch in your side. Hold for 30 seconds on each side and repeat on the other side.

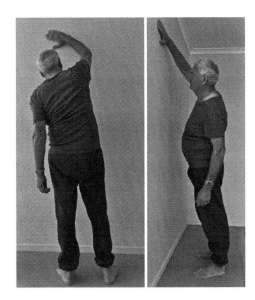

Cool Down: 2 minutes of deep breathing and relaxation

Stand with your back against the wall, breathe deeply and relax your muscles. Keep your breathing in check and practice a breathing exercise (*refer to Chapter four for breathing techniques*) while you clear your mind and focus on mental and physical harmony.

Intermediate:

Warm-up: Same as beginner.

Wall Butterfly Stretch (One minute):

Sit on the floor with your back against the wall and, knees bent, soles of your feet together. Gently press your knees outwards, feeling a stretch in your inner thighs. Hold for one minute.

Wall Neck Stretch (30 seconds on each side):

Stand with your back to the wall, feet hip-width apart. Move your head from one side, bringing your ear towards your shoulder. Place your hand on the opposite side of your head and gently guide it further without forcing. Hold for 30 seconds on each side.

Wall Seated Forward Bend (One minute):

Sit on the floor with your back against the wall and your legs extended. Reach your arms overhead and slowly fold forward, reaching towards your toes or shins. Keep your back straight and feel a stretch in your hamstrings and back. Hold for 30 seconds, then repeat.

Cool down: Same as beginner.

Advanced:

Warm-up: Same as beginner.

Wall Inner Thigh Stretch: (30 seconds on each side, repeat on each side twice)

Lay on your back, bending your legs with feet resting flat on the floor. Cross one ankle over the opposite knee, resting it near your thigh. Press your knee toward the floor, feeling a stretch in your inner thigh.

Wall Wrist Flexor Stretch: (Hold each hand for 30 seconds and repeat four times).

Stand with your back facing the wall, feet hip-width apart. Place your hands flat on the wall, fingers pointing down. Gently lean forward, with your back straight, until you feel a stretch in your forearms and wrists.

Cool down: Same as beginner.

Let's get rid of those aches, shall we? Get exercising as we work on building core strengths in the next chapter.

CHAPTER 3

BUILDING CORE STRENGTHS WITH WALL PILATES

"A strong core is your internal compass, guiding you through life's journey."

Ever wonder why dancers seem to move with effortless grace? The secret lies not in fancy footwork but in a powerhouse hidden beneath the surface – their core. Time, as it passes, can dim the fire within our muscles, making years of bending, lifting, and carrying seem like a distant memory. But what if you could reclaim the power that directs every movement? This is where Wall Pilates comes in with the magic of building your core strength and rediscovering the forgotten power within your centre.

Understanding The Importance of Core Strength for Seniors

Think of your core as the conductor of your orchestra, orchestrating every movement, from reaching for a high shelf to laughing with abandon. Strong core muscles aren't just about sculpted abs (though, who wouldn't welcome that!); they're the silent heroes holding your spine upright, providing balance, and boosting your confidence with every step.

Benefits of Strong Core for Everyday Activities

Here's how a strong core benefits your everyday life:

Ditch the aches and pains: A supportive core helps maintain proper posture, reduces back pain and joint discomfort, and lets you navigate your day efficiently.

Embrace newfound freedom: Strong core muscles act like invisible hands, assisting you in bending, lifting, and carrying, allowing you to reclaim the joys of daily activities without struggle.

Improved balance and stability: Imagine navigating cobblestone streets with confidence! A strong core offers a steady base, diminishing the likelihood of falls and amplifying your sense of stability.

Boost your mood and energy: Feel the spring in your step! Core strength improves circulation and oxygen flow, leaving you feeling revitalised and ready to tackle anything.

Common Strength Myths for Seniors

Our journey towards a more robust core begins by dispelling some common myths often told about seniors and this vital muscle group. Forget the exhausting crunches and rigid planks; Wall Pilates offers a gentler, more sustainable approach.

Myth 1: *"Strong core equals six-pack."* While sculpted abs may be aesthetically pleasing, they're not the sole indicator of core strength. Wall Pilates focuses on strengthening the deeper layers of your abdominal muscles, which are responsible for your stability and everyday movement.

Myth 2: *"Age is a barrier."* Time doesn't have to dictate your core's potential. Wall Pilates exercises are adaptable and cater to all fitness levels, ensuring a safe and effective journey for seniors.

Myth 3: *"No pain, no gain."* Forget the grunting and grimacing! Wall Pilates emphasises mindful movements and deep core engagement, improving strength without unnecessary strain.

Principles of Core Training in Wall Pilates

Stepping into the realm of practical principles, wall Pilates builds core strength through:

Quality over quantity: Gentle, controlled movements with proper form are essential. Listen to your body and avoid pushing yourself to the point of pain. Remember, consistent practice with mindful engagement is more effective than sporadic intense workouts.

Alignment: Posture matters! Gentle stretches and exercises promote a healthy spine and pelvis alignment, creating a solid foundation for core engagement.

Breathing: Breath is the fuel that powers your core. Wall Pilates emphasises synchronised breathing with movement, enhancing oxygen delivery and muscle activation.

The Role of Core Stability in Balance

Think of your core as your body's control centre. When it's solid and stable, it acts like a gyroscope, keeping you upright and balanced.

This is especially important for seniors, as good balance helps prevent falls and maintains independence. Wall Pilates exercises strengthen your core muscles, improve your posture, and enhance proprioception (awareness of your body in space). This means a confident gait, reduced risk of falls, and a newfound freedom of movement.

Incorporating Core Exercises into Daily Routine

Integrating core exercises into your daily routine doesn't require grand gestures or lengthy sessions. Start small, perhaps with simple exercises while brushing your teeth. Consistency is key – even five minutes of mindful engagement can work wonders. Here are some ways to sneak core exercises into your day:

Postural Power: During waiting periods, such as in a line or at the bus stop, activate your core by bringing your belly button towards your spine and standing tall with good posture.

Desk Warrior's Twist: Stuck at your desk? Take a break and perform a gentle spinal twist. Sit tall, place your hands on your knees, and twist your torso slowly to one side, feeling the stretch in your core muscles. Repeat on the other side.

Kitchen Cardio: While washing dishes or prepping dinner, activate your core by tightening your abdominal muscles and bringing your belly button in. This simple act strengthens your deep core, the powerhouse behind every movement.

Stairway Serenade: Climbing stairs? Use them as an opportunity to improve your legs and core. Take each step slowly and deliberately, and stay focused on engaging your abdominal muscles with each step.

These are just a few starting points. You can gradually introduce specific Wall Pilates exercises designed to target your deep core muscles as you progress.

Gradual Progression in Core Strength Training

Building core strength with Wall Pilates is a gradual journey. Each movement strengthens your inner powerhouse, step by step. Forget the days of pushing yourself to the limits.

Start with exercises that engage your core subtly, focusing on proper form and alignment. Simple yet effective movements like wall pelvic tilts and wall slides will awaken your muscles without strain.

As you gain confidence and control, gradually increase the intensity of exercises. Explore variations with minor progressions, adding props like resistance bands or chairs to increase the challenge. Remember, consistency is key!

Tips for Maintaining a Stable Core during Exercises

Here are some additional tips for maintaining a stable core during Wall Pilates exercises:

Visualise your centre: Imagine a ball of energy emanating from your core, radiating strength and control.

Engage your glutes: Don't rely solely on your abdominal muscles. Squeeze your glutes together to stabilise your pelvis further and prevent strain.

Don't hold your breath: Breathe deeply and rhythmically throughout the exercises, ensuring proper oxygen flow to your muscles.

Listen to your body: Pain is a signal, not a badge of honour. Stop or modify any exercise that causes discomfort.

Core Strength Assessment for Seniors

Before embarking on our journey to reclaim inner strength, let's take a moment to listen to your core. This isn't a gruelling test but a gentle exploration of your current capabilities.

Try simple exercises like holding a plank against the wall, performing side planks, or engaging your core while marching in place. Pay attention to how easily you can maintain these positions and identify any areas that feel weak or uncomfortable.

This self-assessment will guide you toward the exercises that will most benefit your unique needs.

Core Strength Maintenance Between Wall Pilates Sessions

While Wall Pilates sessions are your dedicated practice time, maintaining core strength throughout the day is critical.

Take the stairs instead of the elevator, engage your core as you reach for something high, or tighten your abdominal muscles while standing in line. These seemingly small actions weave strands of strength into your daily life.

And remember, movement doesn't need to be strenuous. Even while watching TV or reading a book, gentle stretches like side bends or pelvic tilts can work wonders for your core. Listen to your body and choose movements that feel good, not gruelling.

Core Exercises

For Improved Digestion: Are you feeling out of sync? Gentle twists like Wall Spinal Rotations can stimulate your digestive system, while Wall Leg Lifts can activate abdominal muscles that aid digestion.

For Lower Back Support: Does your lower back whisper complaints? Wall-supported Bridge exercises strengthen your core and glutes, creating a supportive foundation for your spine. You can also explore gentle Wall Cat-Cow stretches for added relief.

For Better Posture: Are you longing for a regal bearing? Standing Tall with Shoulder Rolls lengthens your spine and improves your posture, allowing you to stand tall and radiate confidence. Wall Chest Openers can enhance your upper body posture, creating a harmonious balance.

For a better understanding and explanation, refer to the Exercise List at the end of the chapter or to previous chapters above.

Integrating Core Training with Other Forms of Exercise

Your journey to a strong and vibrant core isn't confined to the gentle embrace of the wall.

Yoga: Flow with the grace of a willow tree as you combine gentle Wall Pilates stretches with the mindful movements of yoga. This harmonious blend strengthens your core while promoting balance and flexibility.

Walking: Turn your daily walks into a core-strengthening adventure! Engage your core muscles as you walk, focusing on drawing your belly button in and maintaining a tall posture. This subtle shift adds an extra layer of workout to your daily routine.

Swimming: Dive into the refreshing world of aquatic exercise. Buoyancy supports your body while allowing for gentle core-engaging movements like flutter kicks and water crunches.

Core Exercises for Pelvic Floor Health

Pelvic Floor Harmony: Don't neglect the hidden conductor! Wall Pilates offers gentle exercises like Kegels and pelvic tilts that strengthen your pelvic floor muscles, improving bladder control and overall pelvic health.

Breathing Beats: Your breath is the rhythm section! Focus on mindful breathing during Wall Pilates exercises to ensure your internal orchestra performs in perfect harmony.

***

Preview of Exercise List in This Chapter

THE EXERCISES BELOW PROVIDE gentle yet effective Wall Pilates movements tailored for seniors, targeting your core muscles with precision and safety. We'll also explore invigorating options for those who want to push their limits, always emphasising mindful movement and listening to your body's unique rhythm.

Be prepared to rediscover the joy of effortless posture, the confidence of an intense centre, and the vibrant possibilities that unfold with each mindful exercise against the wall.

Exercise List

Beginner

Warm Up (two minutes):

Neck Circles: Gently roll your head in a clockwise circle for 30 seconds, followed by an anti-clockwise circle for 30 seconds.

Torso Twists: Place your hand on your hips and rotate your torso to the right and left for 30 seconds.

Hip Circles: Stand with your feet spaced hip-width apart and softly rotate your hips in a left and right circular motion for 30 seconds.

Wall Abdominal Breathing (two minutes):

Sit on the floor with your back against the wall and knees bent. Rest your feet flat on the floor and lengthen your spine towards the ceiling.

Place one hand on your stomach and the other on your chest. Breathe deeply through your nose, feeling your stomach widen and narrow with every inhale and exhale. Imagine your breath filling your core like a balloon.

Continue focusing on your breath, observing its natural rhythm, and feeling your body relax with each exhale. Breathe slowly and evenly, aiming for two minutes of mindful breathing.

Wall Plank with Leg Lifts (10-12 repetitions per leg):

Stand facing the wall, arms bent at shoulder height, elbows aligned with your shoulders, and forearms against the wall. Activate your core muscles and keep your body straight from your head to your heels.

Lift one leg off the floor, keeping your knee bent and foot flexed. Squeeze your glute and hold for five seconds before lowering. Repeat with the other leg.

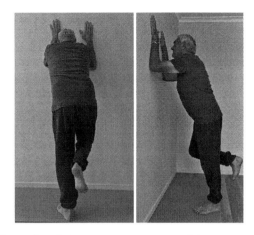

Wall Oblique Crunches (12-15 repetitions per side):

Lay on your back with your knees bent and feet resting flat on the floor. Reach your arms straight towards the ceiling, and press your lower back into the mat. Imagine drawing your navel towards your spine.

Slowly crunch your left arm and right knee towards each other. Rotate your torso diagonally, aiming to bring your elbow towards your thigh.

Feel the squeeze in your oblique as you complete the crunch. Hold for three seconds, then return to the starting position with control.

Repeat the crunch on the other side. Continue alternating sides for 12-15 repetitions per side.

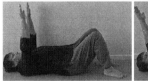 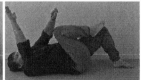

Wall Knee Tucks (10-12 repetitions):

Stand with your back against the wall with your feet hip-width apart. Lean back slightly and touch your tailbone to the wall. Activate your core and keep your back straight.

Raise one knee towards your chest, drawing your navel towards your spine. Hold for three seconds before slowly lowering. Repeat with the other leg for 10 – 12 repetitions.

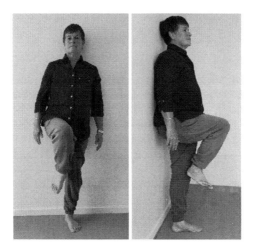

Cool Down: 2 minutes of deep breathing and relaxation

Stand with your back against the wall, breathe deeply and relax your muscles. Keep your breathing in check and practice a breathing exercise (*refer to Chapter four for breathing techniques*) while you clear your mind and focus on mental and physical harmony.

Intermediate

Warm Up: Same as Beginner.

Wall Side Plank (30 seconds per side):

Stand facing a wall with your right hip closest to it. Keep your feet hip-width apart and parallel to each other. Lean onto your right forearm, placing your elbow directly under your shoulder. Engage your core and press your palm firmly into the wall.

Stretch your left arm upward towards the ceiling, keeping it straight, fingers spread. Stack your legs on each other, with your right foot on your left ankle.

Engage your core and squeeze your glutes. Lengthen your entire body in a straight line, forming a diagonal plank from head to heels. Imagine pulling your belly button towards your spine.

Breathe and hold this position for 30 seconds. Maintain good posture, keep your hips level, and avoid letting your body sag towards the wall. Repeat on the other side, holding for another 30 seconds.

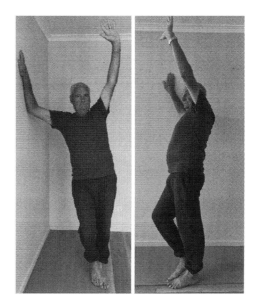

Wall Russian Twists (10-12 repetitions per side):

While seated, with your back against the wall, place your feet flat on the floor and raise your knees to a bending position. Lean back slightly and touch your shoulder blades to the wall. Stretch your arms straight out to the sides.

Activate your core and twist your body to the right, reaching your hands towards the wall on your right side. Breathe in, return to the centre and twist to the left on the exhale.

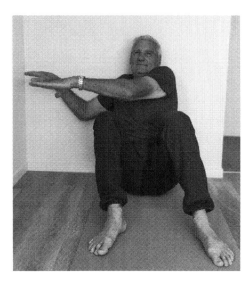

Wall Toe Taps (15-20 repetitions per leg):

Stand with your back on the wall, feet hip-width apart, and arms down by your sides. Keep your core engaged and back straight.

Tap your right heel up and down against the wall, maintaining constant contact. Do 15-20 taps, then switch legs and repeat.

Cool Down: same as beginner

Advanced

Warm Up: Same as Beginner.

Wall Sit (30-60 seconds):

Stand with your back against the wall. Lean back until your tailbone touches the wall, and slide down until your thighs are parallel to the floor (like sitting in an imaginary chair).

Keep your back straight, core engaged, and knees aligned with your ankles. Breathe deeply and evenly. Feel the burn in your quads and glutes. Do this three times, hold for 30 – 60 seconds.

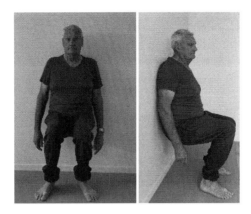

Wall Scissor Kicks (10-12 repetitions per leg):

Lie on your back with your legs extended up the wall and your feet together. Rest your head and shoulders on the ground and engage your core.

Slowly open your legs apart, gliding your heels down the wall until your legs form a diamond shape. Breathe in as you open. Briefly hold the position with control, then slowly bring your legs back together, sliding your heels up the wall and exhaling as you close. Repeat for the desired repetitions.

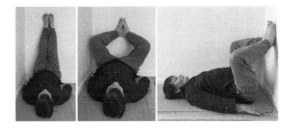

Cool Down: same as beginner

Build your core and improve balance. You should be excited about the next chapter as we tackle pain relief. See you there!

CHAPTER 4

PAIN RELIEF - ALLEVIATING JOINT AND MUSCLE DISCOMFORT

"Pain is not an obstacle; it's a guide."

Feeling like a fragile porcelain doll with aching muscles and inflamed joints? Forget expensive massages and harsh painkillers! Genuine pain relief doesn't have to be a complex melody. Wall Pilates offers a gentle revolution, inviting you to soothe aches, strengthen muscles, and rediscover the freedom of movement with mindful poses and the support of your wall.

Common Joint and Muscle Discomfort in Seniors

The vibrant journey of life can sometimes be accompanied by a subtle counterpoint—discomfort in joints and muscles. This is particularly true for seniors, where years of wear and tear and age-related changes can lead to aches, stiffness, and even inflammation, often concentrated in knees, hips, backs, and shoulders.

Understanding Inflammation and Its Impact

Our bodies are complex ecosystems, and sometimes, the balance within falters. Inflammation is the body's natural reaction to injury or excessive use.

Think of it as a protective wall built around injured tissue, but one that can limit our movement and happiness. Some of the impacts on your life are:

Stiffness and Joint Pain: Chronic inflammation sends pain signals even without injury. This can cause chronic knee, hip, and back stiffness and pain, limiting mobility and daily activities.

Muscle Weakness and Fatigue: Inflammation damages muscle tissue, causing weakness and tiredness. This makes ordinary chores like climbing stairs or carrying groceries difficult, reducing independence and quality of life.

Increased Risk of Falls: Weak muscles and inflexible joints put elders at risk of falling, potentially resulting in fractures and mobility challenges. Inflammation complicates daily life by contributing to both.

Reduced Balance and Coordination: Chronic inflammation can damage nerves and brain function, causing balance and coordination deficits. This can impair walking, increase fall risk, and prevent seniors from enjoying their favourite hobbies.

Negative Impact on Sleep: Inflammation can interrupt sleep patterns, leaving seniors tired and unable to function. Sleep deprivation increases inflammation, which can increase physical and emotional stress.

How Wall Pilates Can Alleviate Discomfort

Forget harsh painkillers and expensive massages. Wall Pilates offers a gentle yet practical path to pain relief. Its mindful movements, supported by the comforting presence of your wall, will help you;

Strengthen muscles: Strong muscles support and protect your joints, reducing strain and inflammation. Wall Pilates exercises gently build strength, creating a supportive foundation for a pain-free life.

Improve flexibility: Stiffness can exacerbate pain, making simple movements a struggle. Wall Pilates stretches—like those discussed in previous chapters—gently increase flexibility, restoring fluidity and ease to your movements.

Reduce inflammation: Concise movement, like the gentle yoga-inspired stretches in Wall Pilates, can reduce inflammation over time. These exercises help with discomfort by encouraging blood flow and promoting tissue repair.

Boost mood and well-being: Moving your body, even when facing pain, releases endorphins, our natural pain relievers. Wall Pilates, focusing on breath and specific movement, promotes physical and emotional well-being, adding a brighter melody to your everyday life.

Specific Wall Pilates Techniques for Pain Reduction

Here are some specific techniques to help your pain:

For knee pain: Gentle movements like wall leg lifts (Chapter one) can strengthen surrounding muscles and reduce pressure on the knee joint.

For hip pain: Wall Side Leg Lifts (*as shown in the exercise list below*) target hip muscles, improving stability and reducing stiffness.

For back pain: Wall Cat-Cow stretches (*Chapter two*) and gentle Wall Pelvic Tilts (*Chapter three*) mobilise the spine, easing tension and promoting flexibility.

For shoulder pain: Wall Arm Circles and Neck Rolls (*Chapter one*) gently improve shoulder mobility and alleviate neck and upper back stiffness.

Tips for Joint-Friendly Wall Pilates

Your body is unique, and Wall Pilates offers a symphony of movements tailored to its specific needs. While enjoying the benefits of strengthening and reliving pain, always listen to your body and prioritise joint-friendliness.

Here are some helpful tips;

Tip 1: *"Listen to your body."* This is your guiding conductor. Stop and modify any exercises that cause discomfort, or take a mindful breath and rest.

Tip 2: *"Start slow and gentle."* Ease into your practice by choosing beginner-friendly exercises like Wall Pelvic Tilts. Build strength and confidence before exploring more challenging movements.

Tip 3: *"Focus on form."* Align your body correctly to distribute weight evenly. Feel free to modify exercises to maintain proper form.

Tip 4: *"Embrace the wall."* Let your personal wall partner offer support and stability. Lean against it for balance in exercises and as a gentle guide.

Tip 5: *"Mindful breathing."* Breathe deeply and rhythmically to oxygenate your muscles and tissues, promoting ease and flexibility. Remember, your breath is the conductor setting the pace for your movements.

Tip 6: *"Listen to your inner voice."* Celebrate even small victories! Each ache soothed, each movement completed with grace, is a note in your progress.

Using Props to Support Joint Health

Sometimes, our joints need a little extra help. Props can help modify exercises, distribute weight, and ensure optimal alignment, especially for those with joint concerns. They can also provide support and comfort during Wall Pilates exercises. Here are a few;

Foam rollers: Place them under your knees or sit on them in seated exercises for added height and support, reducing strain on your lower back and hips.

Straps: Loop them around your feet or ankles for assistance in leg lifts or stretches, providing gentle traction and improving flexibility.

Softballs: Use them between your knees or under your glutes for added stability and proprioception in balance exercises, enhancing joint awareness and control.

Wall Pilates for Arthritis Relief

Arthritis, with its joint pain and stiffness, can seem like a nightmare. But Wall Pilates can be of great help. Specific exercises can manage the symptoms, improve joint mobility, and alleviate pain.

Wall Cat-Cow stretches (*Chapter two*): These gentle movements lubricate your spine and improve flexibility, reducing stiffness and pain in the back and neck.

Wall-side Leg Lifts (*Exercise listed below*): These strengthen hip muscles, providing stability and reducing pressure on arthritic knees.

Wall Leg Circles (*Chapter one*): Gentle circles improve knee joint mobility and circulation, easing stiffness and discomfort.

Listen to your body and modify exercises as needed.

Wall Pilates for Osteoporosis Management

Osteoporosis, with its increased risk of fractures, can make your life seem challenging. However, Wall Pilates offers a gentle yet effective way to manage symptoms and build strength without the strain of high-impact exercises:

Wall Pelvic Tilts (*Chapter three*): These strengthen core muscles, which support and stabilise your spine, reducing the risk of falls and fractures.

Wall Side Plank Variations (*Chapter three*): These modified side planks, supported by the wall, gently strengthen your core and upper body muscles, improving posture and stability.

Prioritise form over force and always listen to your body.

Wall Pilates for Muscular Tension Relief

Muscular tension, like a tangled knot in your body, can restrict movement and cause discomfort. Wall Pilates helps with unknotting tension and restoring ease:

Wall Roll Down (*Chapter one*): These gentle rolls release neck and upper back tension, easing headaches and improving posture.

Wall Arm Circles (*Chapter one*): These gentle circles improve shoulder mobility and loosen tight muscles, reducing stiffness and pain.

Wall Hamstring Stretch (*Chapter one*): This supported stretch gently lengthens hamstrings, relieving tension and improving lower back flexibility.

Wall Pilates for Sciatica Relief

Sciatica pain can feel like a burning or electric shock, and having this all the time can be frustrating and draining. With Wall Pilates exercises, these pains can be eased:

Wall Side Leg Lifts (*Exercise list below*): Your piriformis muscle can be tensed and immobile, contributing to sciatica pain. Wall-side leg Lifts can help release tension and improve flexibility.

Wall Plank (*Chapter one*): A strong core and back support the spine, reducing pressure on the sciatic nerve and easing pain. Wall Plank variations can be adapted for sciatica relief.

Wall Chest Opener (*Exercise list below*): Maintaining proper posture aligns the spine and alleviates pressure on the sciatic nerve. Wall Chest Openers can help improve posture and alleviate pain.

Mindful Movement for Pain Reduction

Embracing gentle, mindful movements throughout your day can transform the pain and aches and reward you with ease.

Morning Flow: Greet the day with gentle stretches. Reach for the sky with your arms, roll your neck like a cat, and side-bend like a swaying willow.

Desk Delights: Break up sitting spells with mini-movements. Roll your shoulders, circle your wrists, and perform seated foot flexes to keep energy flowing.

Kitchen Choreography: Transform daily tasks into graceful dances. Bend and stretch while washing dishes, lift and lower items with intention while cooking, and walk mindfully between tasks.

Evening Tranquility: Wind down with calming movements. Lie on your back, perform gentle knee circles, rock side-to-side like a baby in a cradle, and finish with deep, mindful breaths.

Breathing Techniques for Relaxation and Pain Management

The symphony of pain relief isn't just about movement; it's about harnessing the power of your breath. Here are some specific breathing techniques to integrate with your Wall Pilates practice:

Deep Breathing: Sit or stand comfortably against your wall. Inhale slowly and deeply through your nose, feeling your belly expand gently. Hold for 3-5 seconds. Exhale slowly and thoroughly through your mouth, imagining tension leaving your body with each exhale. Repeat 5-10 times.

Pursed-Lip Breathing: In any Wall Pilates exercise where you feel tension, especially in your neck or shoulders, inhale slowly through your nose. Purse your lips as if about to whistle, and exhale slowly and steadily through pursed lips. Repeat 5-10 times.

Alternate Nostril Breathing: Sit comfortably against your wall with your back straight and feet planted on the floor. Cover your right nostril with your thumb and inhale gently through your left. Close your left nostril with your ring finger and exhale slowly through your right nostril. Proceed to inhale through your right nostril, close it, and exhale through the left nostril. Continue alternating sides for 5-10 cycles.

Rhythmic Breathing: During any wall Pilates exercise, there are prolonged and controlled movements. Synchronise your breath with your movement. For example, inhale as you raise your leg in a Wall Leg Lift (*Chapter 1*) and exhale as you lower it. Maintain a consistent rhythm throughout the exercise for 3-5 times.

Focused Breathing: Lay on your back, feet on the floor, and knees bent. Place one hand on your chest and the other on your belly. Your belly should rise and fall with each inhale and exhale. Breathe deeply and slowly, focusing on calming your mind and body. Do this for 2 minutes.

Addressing Common Misconceptions about Exercise and Pain

Myth 1: *"Pain is Inevitable with Age."* While some discomfort is expected as we age, persistent pain isn't a natural part of aging. Regular, appropriate exercise, such as Wall Pilates, can alleviate and prevent joint and muscle pain.

Myth 2: *"Exercise Causes More Pain."* The right exercises, tailored to individual needs, can reduce pain. Low-impact activities like Wall Pilates enhance flexibility, strengthen muscles, and improve overall mobility without exacerbating discomfort.

Myth 3: *"Rest is the Best Solution for Pain."* Rest is essential, but too much inactivity can worsen the pain. In Wall Pilates, gentle, controlled movements stimulate blood flow, promote healing, and prevent stiffness.

Myth 4: *"Pain Medication is the Only Solution."* While medications have their place, they shouldn't be the sole solution. Exercise can complement medication by addressing the root cause of pain and promoting long-term relief.

Wall Pilates for Better Sleep and Recovery

Incorporating Wall Pilates into your routine can be a transformative practice for improving sleep and overall recovery. Here's how:

Relaxation and Stress Reduction: Wall Pilates exercises often involve controlled movements and mindful breathing, promoting relaxation and reducing stress. A calm mind and relaxed body are conducive to better sleep.

Release of Tension: Many Wall Pilates movements, some of which we have addressed, focus on stretching and releasing muscle tension. This can be beneficial for seniors who experience muscle tightness or discomfort, creating a more comfortable and relaxed state before bedtime.

Mindful Breathing Techniques: As we have mentioned above, Wall Pilates encourages the integration of mindful breathing techniques. Incorporating controlled breathing patterns into your practice can calm the nervous system, promoting a tranquil state that facilitates better sleep.

Improved Circulation: Improved circulation contributes to better nutrient delivery and waste removal in the body, supporting overall recovery during sleep.

Preventing Insomnia: Regular physical activity, such as Wall Pilates, has helped to improve sleep patterns and reduce the risk of insomnia. Pilates can promote relaxation and well-being, contributing to a more restful night's sleep.

Balancing the Nervous System: Wall Pilates has the potential to harmonise the autonomic nervous system, responsible for overseeing vital functions such as heart rate and digestion. A balanced nervous system is associated with improved sleep quality and a more efficient recovery process.

Adapting Wall Pilates for Specific Joint Conditions

Is arthritis acting up? Ditch the high-impact stuff and focus on smooth, flowing movements like wall arm circles. Think of it as painting the air with your arms; it's friendly and accessible. Seated knee lifts are another winner, building strength without stressing your joints. Listen to your body and don't push through pain – there's a difference between feeling the work and feeling ouch!

Osteoporosis has you feeling fragile? We'll build bone density without all the stress. Wall squats (*Chapter 1*) with resistance bands (think light, comfy ones) are your friend, while supported wall push-ups (using a chair for support) can keep those upper body muscles strong. Form is key—think tall spine and engaged core for maximum benefit.

Knee pain got you hobbling? Let's ditch the ouch factor! Wall leg lifts (*Chapter 1*) are your new best friend, strengthening those muscles around your knee without the impact. Side leg lifts, done with minimal extension, can also help.

Nutrition and Hydration for Joint Health

Now, let's talk about feeding those joints from the inside out. Think of your body as a garden – it thrives with the proper nourishment. Here's how to keep your joint at peak form:

Ditch the inflammatory firestarters: Sugar, processed foods, and unhealthy fats can make your joints grumpy. Instead, fill your plate with colourful fruits and veggies, omega-3-rich foods like salmon and flaxseeds, and lean protein sources like chicken or beans.

Hydration is your secret weapon: Water is the magic potion that keeps your joints lubricated and happy. Aim for eight glasses daily, but adjust based on your activity level and climate.

Combining Wall Pilates with Stress-Reduction Strategies

Feeling stressed? We've got some stress-busting tips to help you move with more ease:

Breathe deep, breathe slowly: This simple act calms your nervous system and helps you release tension. Think of it as a mini-vacation for your mind and body.

Meditation magic: Spend a few minutes before or after your workout meditating. Imagine yourself moving freely, pain-free, and relaxed. It's like a mental spa for your joints!

***

Preview of Exercise List in This Chapter

B ELOW ARE SOME ENGAGING exercises to help with your pain relief journey. Easy Wall Pilates to push you out of your comfort zone while still keeping you indoors.

Exercise List

Beginner

Warm Up (two minutes):

Ankle Circles: Rotate your ankles clockwise and counter-clockwise, focusing on feeling the movement in your ankle joints. Repeat ten times in each direction.

Gentle Walking: Walk around for a few minutes, gradually increasing your pace and leg swings. Aim for 30 seconds of light walking.

Dynamic Stretches: Perform gentle dynamic stretches like leg swings, arm swings, and torso twists with controlled movements for a minute.

Wall Squats:

Stand with your back against the wall, about a foot away from it, and your feet hip-width apart. Lean back against the wall and slide down until your thighs are parallel to the floor, forming a 90-degree angle at your knees.

Keep your back straight and core engaged. Relax your shoulders and breathe deeply. Hold for 30-60 seconds, repeat three times.

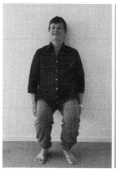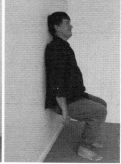

Wall Wrist Extension Stretch:

Stand facing a wall with your feet shoulder-width apart. Your forearms should be flat against the wall, and your fingers should point up. Lean your body slowly forward, keeping your elbows straight and your feet flat on the floor.

Feel the stretch in your wrists and forearms. Hold for 30 seconds, repeat three times.

Wall Child's Pose:

Kneel on the floor with your feet together and sit back on your heels. Extend your arms forward, resting your palms on the wall, and rest your forehead on the floor, with your chest close to your thighs.

Walk your hands out slightly if needed for comfort. Relax your shoulders and breathe deeply. Hold for as long as desired.

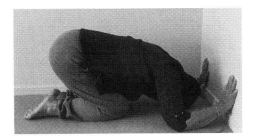

Wall Chest Opener:

Stand facing a wall with your feet shoulder-width apart. Place your forearms flat against the wall at shoulder height, fingers pointing upwards. Lean your chest forward, keeping your back straight and core engaged.

You should feel a gentle stretch in your chest and shoulders. Hold for 30 seconds, repeat three times.

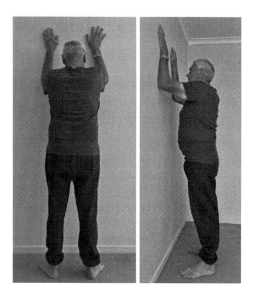

Cool Down: 2 minutes of deep breathing and relaxation

Stand with your back against the wall, breathe deeply and relax your muscles. Keep your breathing in check and practice a breathing exercise (*refer to earlier in this chapter for breathing techniques*) while you clear your mind and focus on mental and physical harmony.

Intermediate:

Warm Up (two minutes): Same as the beginner.

Wall Knee-to-Chest Stretch:

Stand with your back against the wall with your feet hip-width apart. Activate your core and lift one knee towards your chest, bringing your thigh parallel to the floor. Softly press your lower back against the wall.

Maintain the position for 15-30 seconds, then switch legs and repeat the exercise.

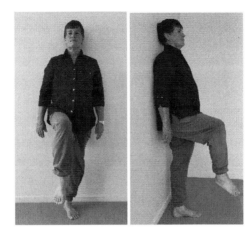

Wall Figure Four Stretch:

Lie on your back with your knees bent and your left foot flat on the wall. Cross your right leg over so that your ankle is over the thigh of your left leg, just above the left knee.

Maintain the position for 15-30 seconds, then switch legs and repeat the exercise.

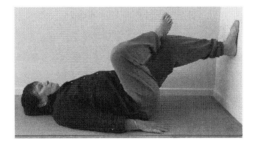

Wall Ankle Circles:

Stand facing the wall, about an inch away from the wall. Lean slightly forward and place your fingertips on the wall for balance.

Make small circles with your right ankle, clockwise and then counter-clockwise. Repeat with your left ankle. Do 10-15 circles in each direction.

Cool down: Same as the beginner.

Advanced:

Warm Up (two minutes): Same as the beginner.

Wall Neck Tilts:

Stand with your back against the wall with your feet hip-width apart and about an inch away from the wall. Gently tilt your head to one side, bringing your ear towards your shoulder.

Hold for 3 - 5 seconds, then slowly return to the center. Repeat ten times on each side.

Wall Wrist Flexor Stretch:

Stand facing a wall with your feet hip-width apart. Place both palms flat against the wall, fingers pointing downwards. Keep your elbow straight and arm extended.

Lean your body forward slowly, keeping your arm straight and heel flat on the floor. You should feel a stretch in your forearm and wrist. Hold for 30 seconds and repeat three – five times.

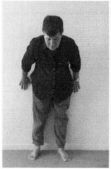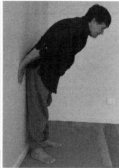

Wall-Seated Spinal Twist:

Sit on the floor with your back against the wall and knees bent. Position your feet firmly on the floor and lift your arms out to the sides.

Activate your core, twist your torso to the right, bring your right hand towards the floor, and rest your left hand on your right thigh. Keep your gaze over your right shoulder.

Feel the stretch in your obliques and lower back. Hold for 30 seconds, then repeat on the other side, repeat three to five times.

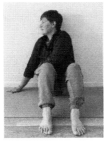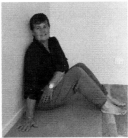

After dealing with pains and improving them, along with healthy joints and bones, we can now focus on increased energy. Let's meet up in the next chapter, where vitality and energy are increased.

CHAPTER 5

GAINING VITALITY THROUGH INCREASED ENERGY

"Energy is the currency of vitality."

Are you feeling bogged down by fatigue? It's time to break free and rediscover the vibrant life you deserve. Imagine waking up each day feeling energised, ready to tackle anything life throws your way, and not feeling drained by the energy of your grandkids or just by the thought of getting up to get that cup of water or coffee. Well, it's your lucky day then because, in this chapter, we will discuss getting that fatigue out the window and getting the energy in.

Understanding Energy Levels in Seniors

As we age gently, our energy levels can change on their own. The days of endless youthful bursts are over, and a more complex rhythm has occurred. But vibrant energy is still in reach! Getting your energy back means figuring out what makes you tired and what makes you happy. Some of these are:

Changes in the body: Losing muscle mass and metabolism with age can make you tired.

Sleep patterns: Not getting enough sleep for different reasons can tire you.

Chronic conditions: Health problems that last for a long time can significantly affect your energy levels.

Nutritional choices: Not getting enough nutrients or eating an unbalanced diet can make it harder to make energy.

Stress and worry: Worry and stress that lasts for a long time can drain your mental and physical energy.

These are everyday experiences, and the good news is that many factors contributing to low energy are under control.

Benefits of Exercise for Boosting Energy

Physical activity might seem counterintuitive when feeling low, but it's a potent energy booster. Here's why:

Increased blood flow: Exercise revitalises oxygen and nutrients in your cells.

Improved sleep: Regular physical activity promotes more profound, restorative sleep, energising you during the day.

Mood enhancement: Exercise releases endorphins, natural mood-elevating chemicals that combat fatigue and promote well-being.

Muscle strengthening: Building muscle mass increases your metabolic rate, burns more calories at rest, and boosts overall energy levels.

Reduce Stress: Physical activity is a natural stress reliever, helping you feel calmer and more resilient in the face of daily demands.

The key is finding activities you enjoy, not dread. Walking, swimming, or dancing are great options for us seniors.

How Wall Pilates Enhances Vitality

Wall Pilates offers a unique blend of benefits that are particularly well-suited for seniors seeking to boost energy:

Low-impact: Gentle on joints and bones, minimising stress and risk of injury.

Full-body workout: Improves flexibility, strength, and balance, leading to more efficient movement and reduced fatigue.

Mind-body connection: Focus on breathing and mindful movements to promote relaxation, reduce stress, and combat emotional fatigue.

Improved circulation: Increased blood flow throughout the body delivers oxygen and nutrients, enhancing energy levels.

Increased confidence: Feeling more robust and more mobile can boost self-esteem and motivation, contributing to an overall sense of vitality.

Wall Pilates is a safe and effective way to reduce stress, build strength, and help improve your flexibility, all of which contribute to increased energy.

The Role of Nutrition in Energy Levels

Food is fuel, and your fuel quality directly affects how much energy you have. Nutrition plays a huge role in energy levels that you may or may not know about;

Macronutrient Ensemble: You can get instant energy from carbohydrates (called "glucose"), while protein controls blood sugar and good fats provide long-lasting energy and help your body absorb nutrients. You can eat complex carbs, lean protein, and healthy fats for a smooth energy flow.

Micronutrient Co-conductors: Antioxidants, vitamins, and minerals work with enzymes to make chemical processes easier, turning food into energy. To get these essential micronutrients, eat foods like whole grains, colourful fruits and veggies, and dairy.

Blood Sugar Stability is Key: Sugary drinks and processed foods cause your blood sugar to rise and fall, which throws off your energy balance. To keep your energy level steady all day, choose well-balanced meals and snacks with protein, healthy fats, and complex carbs.

Hydration Strategies for Increased Energy

Carry a reusable water bottle: Readily available water encourages you to sip throughout the day.

Set reminders: Use phone apps or alarms to prompt yourself to drink regularly.

Flavour your water: Add slices of cucumber, lemon, mint, or berries for a refreshing twist.

Choose hydrating foods: Include fruits and vegetables with high water content, like watermelon, cucumber, and leafy greens.

Breathing Techniques for Energy Boosting

Deep diaphragmatic breathing (refer to chapter four): This rhythmic breathing technique promotes oxygen intake and relaxation, reducing stress and fatigue and energising you.

Alternate nostril breathing (chapter refer to chapter four): balances the nervous system and improves circulation, offering a quick energy boost when needed.

Visualisation techniques: Combine breathing with visualisation of energetic colours or peaceful landscapes to enhance your energy levels and overall well-being.

Wall Pilates for Improved Lung Capacity

Did you know your lungs play a crucial role in energy production? Wall Pilates can help!

Diaphragmatic Breathing Focus: Many Wall Pilates exercises emphasise deep, diaphragmatic breathing, promoting efficient oxygen intake and improved lung capacity. This translates to more energy at the cellular level and a decrease in fatigue.

Posture Matters: Wall Pilates helps correct slouching and strengthens core muscles, leading to better spine alignment and improved lung function. This allows you to take deeper breaths and utilise more oxygen.

Increased Circulation: Regular Wall Pilates practice improves blood flow throughout the body, including the lungs, enhancing oxygen delivery and maximising energy production.

Wall Pilates for Enhanced Endurance

Endurance isn't just about running marathons; it's about having the energy to tackle daily activities. Wall Pilates can help enhance your endurance for all that strenuous work; how? Here's how;

Muscular Strength & Stamina: Wall Pilates exercises target various muscle groups, building strength and endurance, allowing you to have more energy to perform daily tasks with less fatigue and more energy.

Improved Coordination & Efficiency: By increasing body awareness and control, Wall Pilates helps you move more efficiently, reducing wasted energy and allowing you to do more for longer.

Mental Toughness: Mindful movement through Wall Pilates builds mental focus and resilience, helping you overcome fatigue and maintain energy levels during more extended activities.

Interval Training with Wall Pilates

Elevate your Pilates routine by incorporating interval training (interval training is a type of exercise involving several workouts followed by a short rest) against the wall. Alternate between periods of controlled, focused exercises and short bursts of higher-intensity movements. For example, while doing a simple wall pilates exercise, you could add some Jumping Jacks or High Knees (*refer to the exercise list below*), then take a break and continue with your wall pilates.

Burst of energy, sustained benefits: Interweave short bursts of high-intensity Wall Pilates exercises with recovery periods. This boosts heart rate and metabolism, increasing energy expenditure after a workout.

Adaptable for all levels: Start with low-intensity intervals and gradually increase intensity or duration as you build fitness. Modify exercises as needed to ensure safe and practical training.

Time-efficient energy boost: Short, high-intensity sessions are perfect for busy schedules. A 20-minute interval training session can have comparable benefits to a longer traditional workout.

Incorporating Fun and Enjoyable Elements in Wall Pilates

Would you get bored while engaging in your Wall Pilates exercise? Well, it doesn't have to be so. Making Wall Pilates enjoyable enhances motivation and creates a lighthearted approach to fitness, fostering a sustainable and enjoyable exercise routine. So go ahead and;

Turn up the tunes: Choose music that motivates and inspires you. Upbeat tempos can energise your practice, while calming melodies can enhance relaxation.

Partner up or join a class: Working out with others adds a social element, making exercise more enjoyable and potentially fostering accountability.

Embrace creativity: Explore different variations of exercises, invent your own modifications, and add props like light resistance bands or weights.

Celebrate small victories: Acknowledge your progress, no matter how small. Celebrate milestones and reward yourself for sticking with your practice.

Mindful Eating for Sustained Energy

Getting the energy with wall pilates isn't a hundred per cent enough; you need food to keep that energy, and this is how you can do so;

Eat with awareness: Savor your food, focusing on taste, texture, and the act of eating itself. This promotes mindful choices and prevents mindless overeating.

Plan your meals and snacks: Having nutritious options readily available can help you avoid impulsive, unhealthy decisions. Pack snacks for on-the-go and plan balanced meals around complex carbs, lean protein, and healthy fats.

Listen to your body: Eat intuitively, recognising hunger and fullness cues. Aim to focus on nourishing your body and avoid diets for sustained energy, not deprivation.

Hydrate wisely: Water is essential for energy production and digestion. Aim for 8-10 glasses daily, and adjust based on activity level and climate.

Adapting Wall Pilates for Different Times of the Day

Morning: To kickstart your day, opt for energising exercises. These include invigorating stretches, light cardio movements like wall walking (holding the wall and taking light steps, one foot in front of the other), and core strengthening exercises (*refer to chapter three*).

Afternoon: Focus on improving and reducing fatigue. Gentle stretches (*refer to chapter one*), deep breathing exercises, and seated core work can help combat the afternoon slump.

Evening: Wind down and prepare for sleep with calming movements. Include slow stretches, relaxation poses like child's pose against the wall (*refer to chapter four*), and mindful breathing exercises.

***

Preview of Exercise List in This Chapter

NOW, LET'S INCREASE THAT energy and vitality with the friendly exercises below.

Exercise List

Beginner

Warm Up (two minutes):

Leg Swings: Swing each leg forward and backward 10-15 times with a hand on the wall for stability. This is to improve hip flexibility and activate your leg muscles.

Dynamic Stretches: Stretch your arms, legs, and torso with dynamic movements like arm swings (left to right), leg swings(forward and backward), and torso twists (left to right) for 15-20 seconds each. Do this for one minute.

Wall Mountain Pose:

Stand back against a wall with your feet hip-width apart and about an inch away from the wall. Engage your core muscles and gently press the lower part of your back against the wall.

Maintain an upright posture with your shoulders relaxed and lowered, and let your arms hang naturally at your sides. Keep your gaze straight ahead. Hold for 30 seconds to one minute.

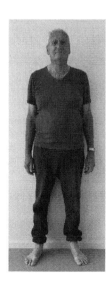

Wall Downward Dog:

Stand facing the wall, about three feet away. Lean down and place your hands on the wall. The ideal position is to create an upside-down "L" shape with your torso and legs.

Push your hands to the wall, draw your hips back, and lightly draw the navel to the spine, softly engaging the core.

Your arms should be level with your ears. Keep your back straight and your core engaged. Gaze down towards your heels. Hold for a minute.

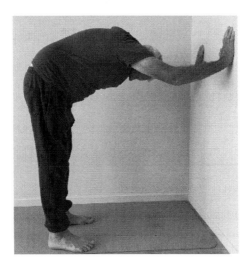

Wall Jumping Jacks:

Stand facing a wall with your feet hip-width apart and arms at your sides. Jump slightly, raising your arms overhead and spreading your legs apart.

Simultaneously, tap your fingertips on the wall in front of you. Lowering your arms, jump back to the starting position, and bring your legs together.

Repeat for 30-60 seconds at a comfortable pace.

Wall High Knees:

Stand with your back to the wall with your feet hip-width apart. Run in place, bringing your knees high towards your chest with each step.

Maintain a tall posture and keep your core engaged. Repeat for 30-60 seconds at a comfortable pace.

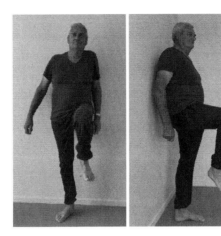

Cool Down:

Gentle Walking: Wind down with one minute of easy walking, calming your breath and body.

Hamstring Stretches: Stand in front of the wall, allowing one hand to lightly touch it for stability. Step backward with one leg, ensuring your heel remains grounded. Lean forward from your hips while maintaining a straight back until you sense a mild stretch in your hamstring. Maintain this position for 30 seconds, then alternate legs.

Intermediate

Warm Up (two minutes): Same as beginner.

Wall Leg Swings:

Stand with your side facing a wall with your feet hip-width apart and about an inch away from the wall. Place your hands flat on the wall for balance.

Swing one leg forward and back, keeping your leg straight and core engaged. Avoid using momentum; focus on controlled movements. Repeat 10-15 swings per leg.

Wall Marching in Place:

Stand with your back against a wall with your feet shoulder-width apart. March in place, bringing your knees high towards your chest at a 90-degree angle.

Keep your back straight and core engaged. Maintain a steady pace for 30-60 seconds.

Wall Arm Raises:

Stand facing a wall with your feet hip-width apart. Place your hands flat on the wall at shoulder height, fingers pointing upwards.

Slowly raise your arms overhead, pressing your palms firmly into the wall. Lower your arms back down to the starting position with control. Repeat 10-15 times

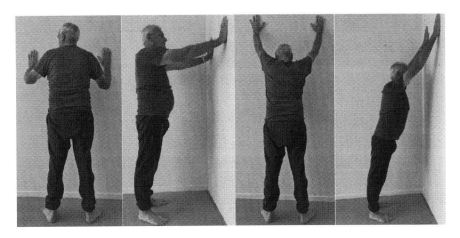

Wall Toe Taps:

Stand facing a wall with your feet hip-width apart and about an inch away from the wall. Standing on your heels, quickly tap your toes against the wall, alternating feet.

Keep your core engaged and maintain a balanced posture. Continue for 30-60 seconds at a fast pace.

Cool Down: Same as beginner.

Advanced

Warm Up (two minutes): Same as beginner.

Wall Side Leg Lifts:

Stand beside a wall with your right side towards it. Place your right hand flat on the wall for balance.

Lift your left leg straight out to the side, keeping your leg parallel to the floor. Lower your leg back down slowly and with control. Repeat 10-15 repetitions per leg.

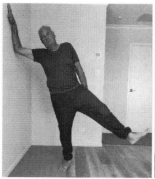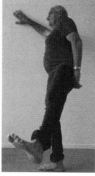

Wall Marching With Arm Circles:

Stand back against a wall with your feet shoulder-width apart and about an inch away from the wall. Engage your core and maintain good posture with your back straight and shoulders relaxed.

Begin marching in place by lifting your knees to a 90-degree angle with each step. Alternate legs in a steady rhythm.

Simultaneously, start small arm circles in forward or backward direction (you can alternate directions with each set). Keep your arms extended to the sides at shoulder level.

Focus on coordinating your leg movements with the arm circles, ensuring both motions flow smoothly. Continue marching and circling your arms for 30 seconds to 1 minute, gradually increasing the intensity as you feel comfortable.

Cool Down: Same as beginner.

You should rest assured that you would not be feeling bogged down by fatigue anymore or as regular, and lifting those grandkids could turn out to be your next favourite thing. Get that energy up, and we'll meet in the next chapter as we foster holistic well-being.

CHAPTER 6

FOSTERING HOLISTIC WELL-BEING THROUGH WALL PILATES

"True well-being is found in the alignment of heart, mind, and body."

Have you ever imagined a practice that strengthens your body, invigorates your mind, and uplifts your spirit? Wall Pilates practice goes beyond stretching and strengthening muscles – it nourishes your mind, soul, and overall well-being in ways you might not expect. The benefits extend far beyond the physical. No matter your fitness level, this chapter invites you to explore the fun of how Wall Pilates can boost your mood, sharpen your memory, and cultivate a sense of inner peace, leading to a new level of life satisfaction and a vibrant embrace of your golden years.

Exploring the Mind-Body Connection in Wall Pilates

We've all heard the saying "mind over matter," but have you ever experienced it firsthand? Wall Pilates offers a unique opportunity to explore the powerful connection between your physical body and your mental and emotional well-being. As you move your body through gentle, controlled exercises, you'll engage your mind in conscious awareness of breath, posture, and movement. This focus fosters a sense of calm and presence, reducing stress and anxiety while enhancing your mood and overall outlook.

Think of it as a dance between your body and your mind. Strengthening your core muscles builds confidence. You improve your balance and gain physical and emotional stability. Releasing tension through mindful stretches experiences inner peace and mental clarity. This link between things makes Wall Pilates such a powerful tool for health in every way.

Benefits of Holistic Well-being for Seniors

Putting our overall health first is even more critical as we age. Wall Pilates focuses on different parts of health and wellness and has many benefits for seniors, including:

Physical:

Improved strength, flexibility, and balance reduce falls and injury risk.

Enhanced joint mobility and pain reduction, allowing for greater independence and daily activities.

Increased bone density, potentially mitigating the risk of osteoporosis.

Mental:

Reduced stress and anxiety, promoting a sense of calm and relaxation.

Improved mood and sense of well-being, combating depression and loneliness.

Enhanced cognitive function, including memory, focus, and concentration.

Emotional:

Increased self-confidence and self-esteem, fostering a positive outlook on life.

Improved sleep quality, leading to increased energy and vitality.

Greater sense of community and connection, primarily through group classes.

Integrating Mindfulness into Pilates Practice

Mindfulness is the act of focusing on the here and now. This is being aware of your thoughts, feelings, and body sensations without getting caught up. Integrating mindfulness into your Wall Pilates practice enhances its benefits:

Set your intention: Before starting, take a moment to set a positive intention for your practice, whether it's improving flexibility, feeling calm, or simply enjoying the movement.

Focus on your breath: Breathe deeply and rhythmically, feeling the rise and fall of your chest and abdomen; notice the sensations of each inhale and exhale.

Embrace present-moment awareness: As you move, pay attention to your body's sensations, the feeling of your feet on the floor, and the stretch in your muscles. Avoid dwelling on the past or future; simply be present.

Accept and release: If your mind wanders, acknowledge it gently and bring your attention back to the present moment. Don't judge yourself; release distractions and return to your movements and breath.

Mindful Breathing Techniques in Wall Pilates

Your breath is your anchor in mindful movement. By using specific breathing techniques, you can further enhance the mind-body connection and reap its benefits:

Deep diaphragmatic breathing: Breathe deeply into your belly, expanding your diaphragm rather than your chest. This promotes relaxation and oxygenates your body.

Alternate nostril breathing: Close one nostril, inhale, hold, then exhale through the other nostril. Repeat on the other side. This calms the mind and balances the nervous system.

Box breathing: Inhale for a count of four, hold for four, exhale for four, and hold for four. Repeat this cycle, focusing on your breath and the present moment.

Experiment with different techniques to find what works best for you. The key is to be gentle, patient, and present in your breath.

Connecting Physical and Mental Well-being

The body is more than just muscles and bones; it's an intricate ensemble of systems that work together to keep us physically, mentally, and emotionally healthy. Wall Pilates is good for your body because it makes you stronger, more flexible, and more balanced. It also positively affects your whole being, making you feel more balanced.

The Mind-Body Link: Our bodies and minds are intricately intertwined. Physical activity releases endorphins, natural mood boosters that combat stress and anxiety. Wall Pilates further amplifies this effect by focusing on controlled movements and mindful breathing. As you move with intention and awareness, your mind quiets, leaving space for clarity and focus.

Building Resilience: Regular Wall Pilates practice strengthens your body, improving balance, flexibility, and coordination. This newfound physical confidence translates into mental resilience. You feel more empowered to tackle challenges, navigate daily life quickly, and bounce back from setbacks with a positive outlook.

Stress Reduction and Improved Sleep: Gentle stretching and controlled movements in Wall Pilates will help melt away tension, leaving you feeling relaxed and rejuvenated. This translates to better sleep quality, crucial for cognitive function and emotional well-being. As you drift off to sleep, you carry the calmness cultivated in your practice, promoting a peaceful slumber and a refreshed start to the day.

Emotional Benefits of Regular Wall Pilates Practice

The emotional benefits of Wall Pilates go beyond simply feeling good. Here's how this practice can nurture your emotional well-being:

Reduced stress and anxiety: As mentioned earlier, Wall Pilates' calming effect on the nervous system reduces stress and anxiety. This can lead to a greater sense of maintaining stability and strength in the face of adversity.

Improved sleep quality: Chronic stress and anxiety often disrupt sleep. With its stress-reducing and relaxation techniques, Wall Pilates can help you fall asleep faster and sleep more soundly, leading to improved mood and energy levels throughout the day.

Increased social connection: Joining a Wall Pilates class or practising with friends can provide a sense of belonging and social connection. This is especially important for seniors who might be facing isolation or loneliness.

Empowerment and self-efficacy: Mastering new movements and feeling stronger in your body can be incredibly empowering. This confidence can spill over into other areas of life, leading to a more positive and proactive approach to challenges.

Incorporating Relaxation Techniques in Wall Pilates

Below are some ways you can add relaxation to your wall pilates journey;

Deep breathing: Throughout your exercise routine, focus on mindful deep breathing. Inhale through your nose slowly, feeling your belly expand, and exhale slowly through your mouth. This calms your nervous system and enhances relaxation.

Progressive muscle relaxation: Tense and release different muscle groups individually, focusing on relaxation spreading through your body.

Guided visualisations: Imagine yourself in a peaceful place surrounded by calming sights and sounds. This visualisation technique can further deepen your relaxation and reduce stress.

Meditation: Before or after your practice, spend a few minutes in quiet meditation. Focus on your breath and observe your thoughts. This practice cultivates inner peace and awareness.

Mindful Walking and Movement Meditation

Wall Pilates isn't just about static exercises. Incorporating mindful walking with gentle arm movements can be a form of moving meditation.

Walk as if on clouds: Incorporate mindful walking with Wall Pilates. Pay attention to the sensations in your feet, the rhythm of your breath, and the world around you. This simple practice reduces stress and anxiety while promoting present-moment awareness.

Move with intention and breathe easily: Integrate basic Wall Pilates exercises into your walks. Perform arm circles, gentle stretches, or leg raises while consciously connecting your breath to your movement. This creates a moving meditation, uniting body and mind for deep relaxation.

Mindful Eating and Nutrition for Overall Health

Imagine fuel that powers your body, uplifts your mood, and sharpens your mind. That's the magic of mindful eating and intentional nutrition! You can explore the connection between mindful eating and wall pilates by having;

Conscious food choices: Choosing whole, unprocessed foods rich in nutrients like fruits, vegetables, and lean protein provides your body with strength, energy, and cognitive function.

The gut-brain connection: Did you know gut bacteria play a crucial role in your mood and mental well-being? Incorporating fermented foods, probiotics, and prebiotics into your diet nourishes your gut microbiome, positively impacting your stress levels, anxiety, and overall well-being.

Mindful eating practices: Paying attention to your hunger cues, savouring each bite, and avoiding distractions while eating can promote healthy digestion, reduce stress-induced eating, and improve your overall relationship with food.

Personalised nutrition: Understanding your individual needs and potential dietary limitations is critical to optimising your energy levels, cognitive function, and overall well-being through mindful eating.

Mindfulness Practices for Improved Sleep

For physical and mental recovery, you need to get enough restful sleep. Wall Pilates can help, but these mindfulness techniques might help you sleep better:

Mindful Breathing: Practice deep, rhythmic breathing exercises learned in Wall Pilates before bed. This calms the mind and prepares your body for sleep.

Improved body awareness: Mindfulness exercises can help you identify and release physical tension, creating a more relaxed state conducive to deeper sleep.

Establishing a relaxing bedtime routine: Integrating mindful breathing and gentle stretches into your pre-sleep routine can signal to your body that it's time to wind down, promoting better sleep quality.

Exploring the Role of Laughter in Holistic Well-being

Laughter isn't just fun; it's a powerful medicine for both body and mind.

Laughter is the best medicine. Laughter produces endorphins, which are natural mood boosters that lower stress, improve circulation, and even strengthen the immune system. Sharing a laugh with a friend in Wall Pilates class or finding humour in everyday life can make you feel better and make your exercise more fun.

Playfulness is critical: Don't take yourself too seriously! Take advantage of the fun way that Wall Pilates makes movement and discovery. Allow yourself to experiment, try new variations, and even laugh at yourself if you stumble. This fun approach can help you feel less stressed, get more motivated, and enjoy your practice more.

Mindful Journaling for Reflection and Growth

Journaling is a powerful tool for self-reflection and growth. Combined with your Wall Pilates practice, it becomes a holistic approach to understanding your mind-body connection and fostering personal development.

Documenting Your Journey: Track your physical and emotional progress through journaling. Record how you feel before and after your practice, noting any mood, energy levels, or mindset changes.

Reflecting on Connections: Use journaling to explore the connection between your physical movements and your emotional state. Did specific exercises trigger certain feelings? How did your mindfulness practice impact your overall well-being?

Setting Intentions and Goals: Use journaling to set intentions for your practice, both physically and emotionally. Define goals you want to achieve and track your progress, celebrating your successes.

Mind-Body Connection and Improved Immune Function

Taking care of your emotional and mental well-being can positively impact your physical health, including your immune system. Wall Pilates and mindfulness practices can play a significant role in this connection:

Reduced Stress Hormones: Stress weakens the immune system. By managing stress through mindfulness and movement, you can reduce cortisol levels and strengthen your immune response.

Improved Sleep: Both practices promote better sleep quality, which is crucial for immune function. Having adequate sleep allows your body to repair and regenerate, boosting its defences.

Increased Positive Emotions: Positive emotions like joy and gratitude have been linked to improved immune function. The uplifting nature of Wall Pilates and mindfulness can cultivate these emotions, contributing to overall health.

***

Preview of Exercise List in This Chapter

Are you excited to learn more about how Wall Pilates can improve your overall health? This chapter discusses workouts that will not only strengthen your body but also wake you up and make you feel better.

Get ready to learn a carefully chosen set of moves that are good for people of all exercise levels. Whether you've been working out for a long time or are just starting, this list includes adjustments and progressions to ensure your practice is safe and effective.

Exercise List

Beginner

Warm-Up (two minutes):

Neck Rolls: Gently roll your head clockwise and counter-clockwise direction, feeling the stretch in your neck muscles. Repeat five times in each direction; do this for 30 seconds.

Arm Circles: Make small circles with your arms forward and backward, gradually increasing the size of the circles. Repeat ten times in each direction; do this for a minute.

Ankle Circles: Rotate your ankles clockwise and counter-clockwise, focusing on feeling the movement in your ankle joints. Repeat ten times in each direction for 30 seconds.

Wall Mindful Breathing (three minutes):

Stand with your back against a wall, your feet hip-width apart and about an inch away from the wall. Place your hands gently on your belly. Close your eyes if comfortable, or gaze downward softly.

Breathe deeply and slowly through your nose, feeling your belly rise and fall with each inhale and exhale. Focus on the present moment and let go of thoughts or worries for three minutes.

Wall Meditation Pose (two minutes):

Stand with your back against a wall with your feet hip-width apart and about an inch away from the wall. Lean your back gently against the wall, keeping your spine straight.

Close your eyes if comfortable, or gaze downward softly. Focus on your breath and the feeling of your body against the wall for two minutes.

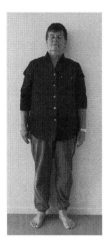

Wall Body Scan Meditation (five minutes):

Lie on the floor with your legs extended and feet against the wall. Close your eyes and focus on your breath.

Slowly bring your attention to different body parts, starting with your toes and moving upwards. Notice any sensations, tightness, or relaxation in each area. Let go of any tension, relax and breathe for five minutes.

Cool-Down (three minutes):

Deep Breathing: Repeat the mindful breathing exercise from the warm-up.

Calf stretch: Lean against the wall with one leg straight and the other bent, pushing your heel towards the wall, then switch legs.

Intermediate

Warm-Up (two minutes): Same as beginner.

Wall Pilates with Soft Music (three minutes):

Perform the Wall Pilates from the beginner level while listening to calming music. Focus on the flow of movement and the connection between your breath and body.

Wall Visualisation Exercise (five minutes):

Sit or stand with your back against a wall and your eyes closed. Imagine performing a specific activity you enjoy, like dancing or playing a sport.

Focus on the sensations and emotions associated with the activity. Feel the joy and confidence of your imagined success, relax and breathe for five minutes.

Cool-Down (three minutes): Same as beginner.

Advanced

Warm-Up (two minutes): Same as beginner.

Wall Relaxation Pose:

Stand with your back against the wall with your hips about an inch away.

Slowly slide down the wall until your back is fully supported, knees bent, and feet flat on the floor, with your bum hanging in the air as if sitting on an invisible chair.

Extend your arms overhead, resting them on the wall or letting them hang naturally at your sides. Close your eyes (optional) and gently release any tension in your body.

Focus on your breath, taking slow, deep inhales and exhales. Stay in this pose for as long as comfortable.

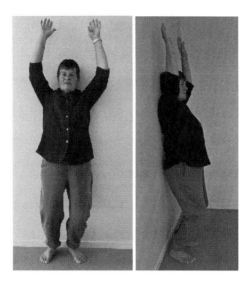

Wall Gratitude Meditation:

Stand with your back against a wall, your feet hip-width apart, and arms at your sides. Close your eyes (optional) and take a few deep breaths to centre yourself.

Bring to mind something you're grateful for, big or small. Imagine placing this gratitude on the wall behind you, visualising it as a warm light or symbol.

Repeat the above, thinking of multiple things you're grateful for and building a wall of gratitude behind you. Feel the warmth and appreciation spreading through your body.

Stay in this mindful state for 5-10 minutes or as long as comfortable.

Cool-Down (three minutes): Same as beginner.

It strengthens your body, invigorates your mind, and uplifts your spirit through these wall pilates exercises and knowledge learned. In the next chapter, we'll discover how to improve balance through wall pilates.

MAKE A DIFFERENCE WITH YOUR REVIEW

UNLOCK THE POWER OF GENEROSITY

"Reclaim Your Vitality, Redefine Later Years with Wall Pilates"

Hey there,

Imagine waking up with the sun, free from morning stiffness. A gentle stretch, a sip of coffee, and you're ready to embrace the day with a smile. Picture yourself effortlessly chasing grandchildren through sunlit parks, joining friends for lively dinners filled with laughter. This isn't a dream, but the life awaiting you beyond this book—a guide to reclaiming your golden years and rediscovering vibrant potential.

Now, let's talk about you. Would you help someone you've never met, even if you never got credit for it?

Who is this person, you ask? They are like you—or, at least, like you used to be—less experienced, wanting to make a difference and needing help but not sure where to look.

Our mission is to make "Quick and Effective Wall Pilates for Seniors" accessible to everyone. Everything we do stems from that mission. And, the only way for us to accomplish that mission is by reaching...well...everyone.

This is where you come in. Most people do, in fact, judge a book by its cover (and its reviews). So here's my ask on behalf of a struggling senior you've never met:

Please help that senior by leaving this book a review.

Your gift costs no money and takes less than 60 seconds to make, but it can change a fellow senior's life forever.

To get that 'feel good' feeling and help this person for real, all you have to do is...and it takes less than 60 seconds...leave a review.

If you feel good about helping a faceless senior, you are my kind of person. Welcome to the club. You're one of us.

I'm even more excited to help you reclaim your vitality and redefine your later years than you can possibly imagine. You'll love the techniques I'll share in the coming chapters.

Thank you from the bottom of my heart. Now, back to our regularly scheduled programming.

Your biggest fan, Laurel Harris

Scan the QR code to leave your review!

CHAPTER 7

WALL PILATES FOR IMPROVED BALANCE

"Balance is the art of standing tall, not despite the winds of change but because of them."

Do you feel unsteady on your feet? Are you worried about falls? Uncover the surprising secret weapon for improved balance—Wall Pilates! Let's reclaim your independence and allow you to embrace a confident-filled life. Wall Pilates offers a gateway to improved balance, empowering you to conquer stairs, enjoy walks, and live life to the fullest.

Understanding the Role of Balance in Aging

Now, seniors, balance is the body's ability to maintain its centre of gravity, ensuring stability and preventing falls. It is necessary for regular activities such as walking, climbing stairs, reaching for objects, and navigating uneven terrain. Balance, which we sometimes take for granted in our youth, becomes more critical as we age. It affects our daily lives, freedom, and overall well-being.

Changes in vision, inner ear function, muscle strength, and the nervous system can all contribute to balance issues as we age. These challenges can lead to falls, which are a serious concern for seniors and can affect our confidence, mobility, and quality of life.

Benefits of Improved Balance for Seniors

Fortunately, there's good news! By prioritising balance exercises like Wall Pilates, you can reap numerous benefits:

Reduced risk of falls: Improved balance translates to a significant decrease in fall risk, protecting you from potential injuries and the associated emotional toll.

Enhanced independence: Maintaining good balance empowers you to confidently navigate daily activities, increasing your autonomy and overall well-being.

Improved physical function: Walking, climbing stairs, and reaching for objects become more accessible and safer with better balance.

Boosted confidence: Knowing you can move with stability and ease fosters a sense of confidence, allowing you to engage in life more fully.

Reduced fear of falling: The constant fear of falling can be debilitating. Wall Pilates can help you overcome this fear, promoting a more active and enjoyable lifestyle.

Common Balance Challenges in Aging Adults

Several specific challenges contribute to balance issues in older adults:

Postural instability: Difficulty maintaining an upright posture while standing or moving.

Weakness in particular muscle groups: Core weakness, particularly in the abdomen and back, is a significant contributor.

Gait and balance disorders: Issues like Parkinson's disease or stroke can significantly impact balance.

Fear of falling can decrease activity and weaken muscles essential for balance.

How Wall Pilates Enhances Balance

Wall Pilates offers a unique approach to improving balance, addressing the root causes through safe and effective exercises:

Strengthening key muscle groups: Targets core, leg, and hip muscles, crucial for stability and posture.

Improving flexibility: Gentle stretches enhance the range of motion, allowing for better adaptation to uneven surfaces.

Neuromuscular training: Exercises challenge the nervous system to react quickly and efficiently to balance challenges.

Fall prevention strategies: Specific exercises mimic real-life situations, teaching your body how to react and recover from potential stumbles.

Mind-body connection: The focus on breath and awareness improves proprioception, your body's sense of position and movement.

Incorporating Balance Exercises into Daily Routine

Start small and integrate balance exercises into your daily routine seamlessly. Here are some ideas:

Brush your teeth: Stand on one leg while brushing, briefly increasing the challenge by closing your eyes.

Do the dishes: Stand on one leg or squat while loading or unloading the dishwasher, holding onto the counter for support if needed.

Take the stairs: Alternate leading with different legs when climbing stairs, gradually increasing the number of steps without using the handrail.

Make it playful: Turn balance exercises into games. Try standing on one leg with a friend or a family member while throwing and catching a ball.

Wall Pilates for Fall Prevention

Many Wall Pilates exercises utilise the wall for support, providing a safe and controlled environment to challenge your balance without fear of falling. Here are some examples tailored to reduce and prevent falls:

Wall heel slides:

Lie on your back, bend your right leg, and place the sole of your foot against the wall. Extend your right leg up the wall with your heel against the wall. Slowly bend your knee and slide your heel down as far as possible.

Hold this position for 20 seconds. Repeat with your left leg. Do this for three minutes.

Wall side squats:

Stand sideways with your hip against the wall and your feet shoulder-width apart. Slowly lower yourself into a squat while keeping your side against the wall. Hold this position for 20 seconds.

Press through your heels to return to standing. Do this for three minutes.

Single-leg wall raises:

Stand facing the wall with one hand lightly placed on it for support. Lift one leg behind you, keeping it straight and parallel to the floor.

Hold for 20 seconds before returning to the starting position. Repeat with the other leg. Alternate legs for two minutes.

Gradual Progression in Balance Training

Start with more straightforward exercises and gradually increase difficulty as you progress. Here are some tips:

Increase repetitions and sets: As you get stronger, do more repetitions of each exercise or add more sets to your routine.

Shorten rest periods: As your endurance improves, decrease the rest time between sets.

Challenge your stability: Once you master an exercise, try it with your eyes closed, standing on an unstable surface (like a pillow), or holding lighter weights.

Listen to your body: Don't push yourself too hard. Consult your doctor if you feel pain or dizziness, and stop immediately.

Tips for Maintaining Stable Balance during Exercises

Keeping your balance during workouts is essential for getting the most out of them and lowering your risk of getting hurt. To help you stay calm and grounded during your workout, here are some essential tips:

Tip 1: *"Engage your core."* A strong core is essential for balance. During each exercise, focus on pulling your belly button towards your spine.

Tip 2: *"Keep your feet flat and grounded."* Distribute your weight evenly across your entire foot for better stability.

Tip 3: *"Focus on a fixed point."* Look at a stable object before you to help maintain your balance.

Tip 4: *"Breathe deeply and steadily."* Avoid holding your breath, as this can make you feel lightheaded.

Balance Assessment for Seniors

Before diving into exercises, it's crucial to understand your current balance level. A simple self-assessment can help you tailor your Wall Pilates practice for maximum impact. Try these tests:

One-leg stand: Stand near a wall for support, lift one leg off the ground, and hold for as long as possible. Repeat on the other side.

Timed Up and Go: Time yourself as you move from a standing position to a seated position, walk three meters, turn around, walk back, and sit again.

Reach test: Sit on a chair and reach forward as far as possible without falling off. Measure the distance.

Nutrition and Hydration for Optimal Balance

The proper nutrients play a crucial role in balance. Focus on:

Lean protein: Builds and maintains muscle mass, essential for balance and stability.

Whole grains: Provide sustained energy and support nervous system function, which is crucial for coordination.

Fruits and vegetables are rich in vitamins and minerals, including calcium and vitamin D, which are essential for bone health.

Healthy fats: Support nerve function and contribute to overall health, indirectly impacting balance.

Balance Exercises for Specific Movement Patterns

Stair mastery: Exercises like single-leg wall squats, step-ups with wall support, and heel-toe walking while facing the wall target the specific muscles and coordination needed for safe stair climbing.

Walking confidently: Improve gait stability and prevent falls with exercises like side leg raises against the wall, alternating heel taps on the wall, and single-leg balancing with eyes closed (while holding onto the wall for safety).

Reaching and bending: Enhance everyday activities like picking up objects or gardening with exercises like wall push-ups on various heights, controlled overhead reaches while standing with wall support, and single-leg deadlifts facing the wall.

Wall Pilates for Enhanced Coordination

Coordination goes hand in hand with balance. Wall Pilates exercises can help:

Eye-hand coordination: Practice throwing and catching a ball while standing against the wall, focusing on smooth movements and visual tracking.

Hand-foot coordination: Challenge yourself with exercises like alternating leg lifts while tapping the opposite hand on the wall, increasing coordination and cognitive function.

Multitasking: Combine balance and cognitive challenges by reciting numbers or colours while performing wall squats or single-leg stands, promoting brain-body connection.

Balance Challenges and Solutions

As you progress, consider these challenges:

Reduce wall support: Gradually decrease the amount of wall support you use in your exercises, challenging your balance system further. For example, try three fingers or one instead of a whole palm supporting you on the wall.

Close your eyes: Briefly close your eyes while performing balance exercises to rely on your inner ear and proprioception.

Limited flexibility: Modify exercises to accommodate your range of motion. Use props like rolled towels or cushions for added support. Focus on maintaining good posture and avoid overreaching beyond your comfort limit.

***

Preview of Exercise List in This Chapter

BELOW IS A COMPREHENSIVE range of exercises that equip you, categorised by difficulty level.

Improving your balance is within reach. Embrace the journey with Wall Pilates and reclaim the confidence and freedom to move with joy and independence.

Exercise List

Beginner

Warm-Up (two minutes):

Gentle Marching in Place: Stand with your feet hip-width apart and march in place, keeping your core engaged and lifting your knees to a 90-degree angle. Repeat for a minute.

Arm Circles: Make small circles with your arms forward and backward, ensure your arms are at shoulder height, gradually increasing the size of the circles. Repeat ten times in each direction for a minute.

Wall Single Leg Balance (one minute for each leg):

Stand facing the wall with your feet hip-width apart and about an inch away from the wall. Place one hand gently on the wall for support.

Slowly lift one leg off the ground behind you and hold it straight for a minute. Keep your core activated and your standing leg stable. Repeat with the other leg.

Wall Heel-to-Toe Walk (one minute):

Stand with your side to the wall with your feet hip-width apart and about an inch away from the wall.

Place one hand gently on the wall for support. Carefully lift one heel off the ground and slowly place it in front of your other toes.

Repeat with the other foot, walking heel-to-toe for a minute up and down the wall. Focus on your balance and keeping your core activated.

Wall Tandem Stance (one minute):

Stand facing the wall, feet hip-width apart and about an inch away from the wall. Place one hand gently on the wall for support.

Stand with one foot directly in front of the other, heel-to-toe.

Hold in this position for 30 seconds, keeping your core activated and your body upright. Repeat with the other foot in front.

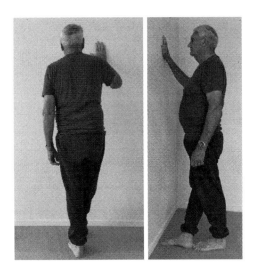

Cool-Down (two minutes):

Deep Breathing: Sit or stand comfortably and take slow, long, deep breaths through your nose and out your mouth. Repeat for 5-10 breaths for a minute.

Gentle Quad Stretch: Hold the wall for support and bring your heel towards your buttocks. Do this for a minute.

Intermediate

Warm-Up (two minutes): Same as beginner.

Wall Clock Reach (10 repetitions on each side):

Stand facing the wall, feet hip-width apart and about an inch away from the wall. Place one hand gently on the wall for support.

Extend your other arm straight out to the side, like the hand of a clock at 3 o'clock. Slowly reach your arm overhead, imagining drawing a circle on the wall like the hand of a clock moving to 12 o'clock.

Return your arm to the side and repeat, tracing the imaginary circle to 9 o'clock. Repeat ten times on each side.

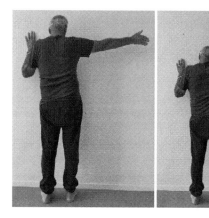

Wall Knee Flexion (10 repetitions on each leg):

Stand with your back on the wall with your feet hip-width apart and about an inch away from the wall. Keep your back straight and core engaged, and slowly bend one knee towards your chest.

Pause for a moment, then slowly straighten your leg back out. Repeat ten times on each leg.

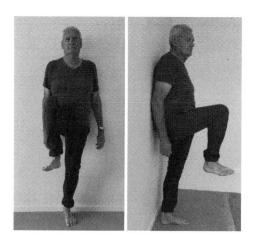

Wall Toe Taps (one minute):

Stand facing the wall, feet hip-width apart and about an inch away from the wall. Place one hand gently on the wall for support.

Tap your toes lightly against the wall, alternating feet as fast as you can comfortably for one minute. Focus on your balance and keeping your core activated.

Cool-Down (two minutes): Same as beginner.

Advanced

Warm-Up (two minutes): Same as beginner.

Wall Lateral Leg Lifts (10 repetitions on each side):

Stand facing the wall with your feet hip-width apart and about an inch away from the wall. Place one hand gently on the wall for support.

Keep your leg straight, and slowly lift one leg out to the side as comfortably as possible. Slowly lower your leg back down. Repeat on each leg ten times.

Wall Figure Eight Exercise (two minutes):

Stand facing the wall with feet hip-width apart and about an inch away. Place one hand gently on the wall for support.

Keeping your leg straight and core engaged, draw small circles in the air with your foot, imagining you're tracing a figure eight. Start slowly and gradually increase the size of the circles.

Continue for 30 seconds on each leg, then repeat.

Wall Sit-to-Stand (10 repetitions):

Stand with your back on a wall. Lower yourself against the wall until your knees reach a 90-degree angle, resembling a seated position in a chair.

Keep your back straight, core engaged, and feet flat on the floor. Push yourself back to standing using your leg muscles and core strength. Repeat ten times.

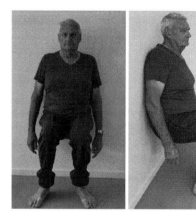

Wall Leg Swing (30 seconds for each leg):

Stand with your side facing the wall with feet hip-width apart and about an inch away. Place one hand gently on the wall for support.

Keep your leg straight and core engaged; swing one leg forward and backward in a controlled manner. Maintain a small swing amplitude and avoid going too high. Continue for 30 seconds, then switch legs and repeat

Cool-Down (two minutes): Same as beginner.

By practising these exercises regularly, you can improve your balance, stability, and overall fitness. After balance is out of the way, we will improve posture in the next chapter.

CHAPTER 8

WALL PILATES FOR BETTER POSTURE

"A strong posture is the foundation for a strong and resilient body."

Hunched shoulders and a sore back? Good Posture is not just about sitting up straight! Imagine feeling taller, stronger, and more confident as you walk. You should be ready to ditch the hunch and embrace a posture that pops. This chapter unlocks the secrets to better posture through the transformative power of Wall Pilates. It offers a unique approach to addressing the root causes of poor posture and transforming your silhouette.

Importance of Good Posture for Seniors

As we age, our bodies go through changes that can impact our posture. Loss of muscle mass, decreased flexibility, and spinal degeneration can lead to slouching, rounded shoulders, and a hunched appearance. But good posture isn't just about aesthetics; it's crucial for maintaining physical and mental well-being. It promotes:

Balance and stability: Strong core muscles and proper alignment significantly reduce the risk of falls, a significant concern for seniors.

Pain relief: Poor posture can lead to aches and strains in the back, neck, and shoulders. Wall Pilates targets these areas to improve alignment and alleviate pain.

Improved breathing: Good posture allows your lungs to expand fully, improving oxygen intake and overall vitality.

Boost in confidence: Standing tall and proud naturally promotes a more positive self-image and enhances confidence.

How Aging Affects Posture

As seniors, several factors contribute to postural changes. Some of these are:

Loss of muscle mass and bone density: Weakened core muscles and decreased bone support make it harder to maintain proper alignment.

Joint stiffness and reduced flexibility: Limited flexibility in the spine and joints can restrict movement and lead to slouching.

Arthritis and other age-related conditions: These can cause pain and discomfort, hindering movement and promoting poor posture.

Benefits of Wall Pilates for Posture Improvement

Wall Pilates offers a unique approach to address these challenges:

Gentle and safe: Ideal for all fitness levels, minimising strain on joints and muscles.

Targeted exercises: Strengthen core muscles and improve flexibility, which is crucial for good posture.

Mindful movement: Promotes awareness of alignment and encourages proper movement patterns.

Functional exercises: Translates improved posture into everyday activities, promoting long-term benefits.

Incorporating Posture Exercises into Daily Life

While Wall Pilates offers a dedicated practice, incorporating simple posture exercises into your daily routine can further enhance the benefits:

Set posture reminders: Use alarms or sticky notes to prompt yourself to stand tall and adjust your posture throughout the day.

Mind your posture while sitting: Sit with your back straight, shoulders relaxed, and feet flat on the floor. Avoid slouching or hunching.

Strengthen your core: Engage your core muscles in everyday activities like walking, standing, and lifting objects.

Stretch regularly: Regular stretches throughout the day improve flexibility and prevent tightness, which contributes to poor posture.

Wall Pilates for Spinal Alignment

Think of your spine as the central pillar of your posture. Wall Pilates uses targeted exercises to address muscle imbalances and strengthen postural muscles, promoting natural alignment from head to toe.

Gentle stretches release tightness in overused muscles, while wall-assisted movements help retrain proper movement patterns. This well-rounded approach fosters a healthy, aligned spine, the foundation for good posture and pain-free movement.

Tips for Maintaining Good Posture during Exercises

Maintaining good posture during Wall Pilates exercises is crucial to maximise benefits and prevent strain. Here are some essential tips:

Engage your core: Every exercise, whether standing or seated, begins with engaging your core muscles. This creates a stable foundation for your spine and prevents slouching.

Maintain a neutral spine: Imagine a straight line running down your spine from your head to your tailbone. Aim to keep this line as straight as possible throughout each exercise.

Focus on alignment, not perfection: Don't get discouraged if your posture isn't perfect initially. Focus on aligning your body correctly and feeling the engagement of your muscles. Over time, your alignment will naturally improve.

Mind your breath: Breathe deeply and naturally throughout each exercise. This keeps your mind focused and oxygenates your muscles, improving their performance and preventing fatigue, which can lead to poor form.

Use the wall as your guide: Lean against the wall for support and feedback. Feel how your body aligns against the wall, and adjust your posture accordingly.

Posture Assessment for Seniors

A personalised posture assessment can help tailor your Wall Pilates practice and address specific concerns. This is how you can assess your posture yourself;

Stand Tall: Stand in front of a mirror in your everyday posture. Check to see if they are slouching or leaning to one side. You should have a straight line from your ears to your hips and legs.

Check Your Balance: Stand without holding onto anything and see if you can stand still for 30 seconds without swaying or needing to grab something. If you feel shaky, your balance might be off.

Watch How You Walk: Take a few steps forward and backward. Pay attention to whether you lean forward or to the side. Your steps should be steady and balanced.

Test Your Strength: Try sitting down and standing up from a chair without using your hands. If you have trouble or feel shaky, it could mean that your muscles are weak.

Check Your Alignment: Sit in a chair and look at your side profile in the mirror. Your shoulders and ears should align, and your back should curve slightly. Avoid slumping forward.

Do a Reach Test: Sit on the edge of a chair and reach for your toes. If you feel pain when you touch them, it could mean that your back or hamstrings are tight.

Posture Maintenance Between Wall Pilates Sessions

While Wall Pilates sessions are crucial, maintaining good posture throughout the day makes all the difference. Implement these simple tips:

Mindful sitting: Avoid slouching by sitting tall with your back against the chair and feet flat on the floor. Regularly check your posture and adjust as needed.

Stretch it out: Counteract the effects of sitting with regular stretches that target tight areas like your chest, shoulders, and hamstrings.

Strengthen your awareness: Engage your core muscles throughout the day, even during simple activities like standing in line or brushing your teeth. This subtle activation helps maintain proper alignment.

Nutrition and Hydration for Optimal Posture

Believe it or not, what you eat and drink plays a role in your posture! Drinking a lot of water throughout the day ensures you stay hydrated. Water keeps your muscles and joints lubricated, improving flexibility and supporting proper alignment.

Also, pay attention to foods high in nutrients and build strong bones and muscles, like dairy products high in calcium and protein-rich foods like lean meats and vegetables.

Posture Exercises for Specific Muscles

Targeted exercises can address specific muscle imbalances that contribute to poor posture.

Tight hamstrings: Wall hamstring stretches (*Chapter one*) improve flexibility and prevent slouching.

Rounded shoulders: Wall angels chest stretches (*Chapter four*) open your chest and strengthen shoulder posture.

Neck pain: Gentle wall neck stretches (*Chapter two*) can ease tension and improve neck posture.

Rounded lower back: Cat-cow stretches (*Chapter two*) for core and glute strengthening.

Wall Pilates for Upper Back Mobility

Tightness in your upper back can lead to slumped shoulders, rounded posture, and pain. This is where Wall Pilates comes in with its gentle stretches and targeted exercises designed to enhance upper back mobility. Cat-cow poses against the wall improve spinal flexibility, while wall chest openers open your chest muscles and promote proper alignment.

This newfound mobility allows you to move easily, reducing tension and discomfort.

Posture Challenges and Solutions

Hunched shoulders, forward head posture, and a protruding belly – these common posture challenges can be addressed through targeted exercises and mindful awareness. Wall Pilates offers solutions to strengthen your upper back muscles and combat rounded shoulders.

Challenge 1: Hunching Shoulders (rounded upper back)

Wall Angels: Stand with your back against the wall, arms outspread and fingertips against the wall. Slowly lift your arms overhead, maintain contact with the wall, and lower back down. (complete three sets of 10 repetitions)

Challenge 2: Forward Head Posture

Chin Tucks: Stand with your back against the wall, head tall and chin slightly lifted. Slowly tuck your chin towards your chest without moving your head forward. Hold for five seconds and release. (complete three sets of 10 tucks)

Wall Neck Stretches: Stand with your back against the wall and slowly tilt your head to one side, ear towards the shoulder. Gently press your hand against the opposite side of your head to deepen the stretch. Hold for 30 seconds and repeat on the other side.

Wall Pilates for Neck and Shoulder Alignment

Neck and shoulder pain often stem from poor posture. Wall Pilates comes to the rescue, with exercises like neck retractions against the wall that strengthen deep neck muscles and alleviate discomfort.

Gentle side neck stretches to release tension, while wall arm circles (*Chapter one*) improve shoulder mobility and alignment. By addressing these key areas, you can experience reduced pain and enjoy greater freedom of movement.

Wall Pilates for Pelvic Tilt Correction

Pelvic tilt refers to the forward or backward tilt of your pelvis. An anterior tilt (excessive forward tilt) can strain your lower back, while a posterior tilt (excessive backward tilt) can limit your range of motion. Wall Pilates addresses both types of imbalances through targeted exercises.

Anterior Tilt Correction: Exercises like wall pelvic tilts (*Chapter three*) strengthen your core and hip extensors, helping to tilt your pelvis back into a neutral position.

Posterior Tilt Correction: Gentle stretches like hamstring and hip flexor stretches (*Chapter two*) improve flexibility and release tightness, contributing to posterior tilt. Wall leg lifts also activate your core and glutes, promoting proper alignment.

Low-Impact Approach: Gentle on your joints, Wall Pilates is beneficial for individuals with pre-existing conditions or limitations. The wall provides stability and support, allowing you to focus on proper form and alignment without undue strain.

Regularly practising these exercises and maintaining proper posture throughout your day will lead to lasting improvements.

Incorporating Ergonomics in Daily Activities

Ergonomics focuses on creating a comfortable and supportive environment for your body during daily activities. The principles of Wall Pilates – mindful movement, core engagement, and proper alignment – can be easily integrated into your routine to prevent discomfort and promote well-being. Here are some examples:

Sitting: Imagine you have a wall behind your back. Sit tall with your shoulders relaxed and core-engaged. Avoid slouching or hunching, and adjust your chair height and support if needed.

Standing: Imagine your body forming a straight line from head to toe. Move your weight evenly on both feet, activate your core gently, and avoid locking your knees. Take breaks to move around and stretch.

Lifting: Engage your core and bend your knees, not your back, when lifting objects. Keep your back straight and avoid twisting. Use your leg muscles for power and lift smoothly.

Sleeping: Select a supportive mattress and pillow that aligns your spine. Sleep on your back or side with a pillow that cradles your neck. Avoid sleeping on your stomach; this can strain your back and neck.

***

Preview of Exercise List in This Chapter

A ND OFF WE GO to the best part of this chapter: exercises tailored to improve posture and broken down into different stages.

Exercise List

Beginner

Warm-Up (two minutes):

Neck Rolls: Gently roll your head clockwise and counterclockwise, feeling the stretch in your neck muscles. Repeat five times in each direction.

Arm Circles: Stretch your arms out to the side at shoulder height. Make small circles forward and backward, gradually increasing the size of the circles. Repeat ten times in each direction.

Wall Shoulder Blade Squeeze (ten repetitions):

Stand with your back to the wall with your feet hip-width apart and about an inch away from the wall. Gently reach your arms back and press your forearms flat against the wall at shoulder height.

Squeeze your shoulder blades together, feeling them move closer towards your spine. Hold for five seconds, then release. Repeat ten times.

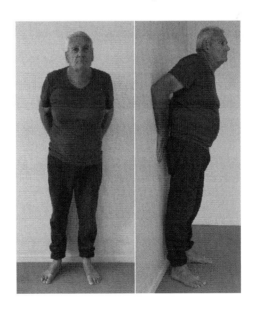

Wall Upper Back Stretch (30 seconds):

Stand facing the wall, feet hip-width apart and about an inch away from the wall. Stretch your arms overhead and place your palms flat against the wall, fingers pointing upwards.

Gently lean your upper body forward, keeping your back straight and core engaged. Feel the stretch in your upper back and shoulders. Hold for 30 seconds.

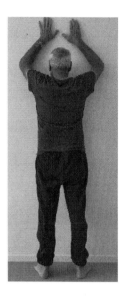

Cool-Down (one minute):

Deep Breathing: Sit or stand comfortably and take deep, slow breaths through your nose and out your mouth. Repeat for 5-10 breaths.

Chest stretch: While standing, clasp your hands behind your back and gently open your chest, pushing your shoulders back.

Intermediate

Warm-Up (two minutes): Same as beginner.

Wall Head Tilt Stretch (30 seconds on each side):

Stand facing the wall, feet hip-width apart and about an inch away from the wall. Place one hand gently on the wall for support.

Tilt your head to one side, bringing your ear down to your shoulder. Gently press your hand against the wall for counter-pressure and feel the stretch in your neck muscles. Hold for 30 seconds, then repeat on the other side.

Wall Forward Neck Flexion (30 seconds):

Stand facing the wall, feet hip-width apart and about an inch away from the wall. Place one hand gently on the wall for support.

Slowly tuck your chin towards your chest, lengthening the back of your neck.

Gently press your hand against the wall for counter-pressure and feel the stretch in the front of your neck. Hold for 30 seconds. Repeat three times.

Wall Thoracic Extension (ten repetitions):

Stand facing the wall with your feet hip-width apart and about an inch away from the wall. Place one hand on the small of your back and the other on the wall at shoulder height.

Gently arch your back backwards, squeezing your shoulder blades together and pushing your chest forward. Hold for ten seconds, then release. Repeat ten times.

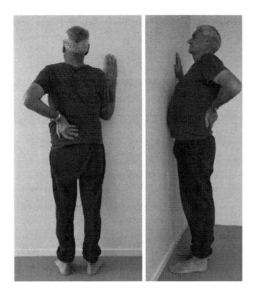

Cool-Down (one minute): Same as beginner.

Advanced

Warm-Up (two minutes): Same as beginner.

Wall Pelvic Tilts (ten repetitions):

Stand with your back against the wall with your feet hip-width apart and about an inch away from the wall. Place your hands on your hips.

Tuck your tailbone under, tilting your pelvis inward to flatten your lower back against the wall. Hold for 15 seconds, then relax and arch your back slightly, tilting your pelvis outward. Repeat ten times.

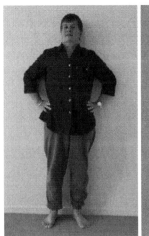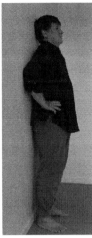

Wall Chest Expansion (ten repetitions):

Stand facing the wall with your feet hip-width apart and about an inch away from the wall. Place your hands flat against the wall at shoulder height, fingers pointing upwards.

Inhale deeply and expand your chest by pushing your chest outward and pressing your hands firmly into the wall. Exhale slowly and release. Repeat ten times.

Wall Seated Posture Corrector (30 seconds):

Stand with your back against the wall, feet flat on the floor. Lower yourself as if seated with knees bent at a 90-degree angle.

Place your hands on your thighs, palms facing down. Gently lengthen your spine and press your lower back into the wall, engaging your core muscles.

Imagine pulling your shoulder blades down and back, opening your chest. Hold for 30 seconds, focusing on maintaining good posture.

Wall Leg Swings (30 seconds per leg):

Stand with your side facing the wall with your feet hip-width apart and about an inch away from the wall. Place one hand gently on the wall for support.

Keep your legs straight, then slowly swing one leg forward and backward in a controlled arc as high as you can comfortably. Focus on using your core and leg muscles to control the swing, not momentum.

To prevent strain, avoid swinging too high or fast. Repeat for 30 seconds on one leg, then switch and repeat on the other.

Cool-Down (one minute): Same as beginner.

Get those hunched shoulders straightened and make your sore back a thing of the past. Wall Pilates is just the thing you need. The magic doesn't stop at better posture but also a happier life, which can be achieved by stress reduction in the next chapter. Ready for the next step? You definitely are.

CHAPTER 9

WALL PILATES FOR STRESS REDUCTION

"In the absence of stress, clarity emerges."

Are you feeling the weight of stress on your shoulders? Is stress just a part of life you have to accept? Well no. Sometimes, stress is inevitable, and carrying it around as a senior isn't something I recommend. You should know that a gentle yet powerful tool for stress reduction is hidden within the world of Wall Pilates. Imagine going through your daily life with more strength and calm.

Dive into the science behind Wall Pilates and discover how mindful movements and gentle exercises can melt away stress, leaving you feeling centred and revitalised.

Understanding Stress and Its Impact on Seniors

Stress, in its various forms, affects everyone. However, seniors can be particularly vulnerable due to life changes, health concerns, financial worries, social isolation and loss. Chronic stress can manifest as emotional strain, sleep disturbances, and even physical ailments. It has the potential to compromise your immune system, contribute to anxiety and depression, and even worsen existing health conditions.

While managing stress effectively is crucial for well-being at any age, it becomes even more important as we mature.

Benefits of Wall Pilates for Stress Reduction

Wall Pilates offers a unique approach to stress management, addressing both physical and mental aspects. Here's how:

Reduced muscle tension: Gentle exercises release built-up tension, easing aches and pains often associated with stress.

Improved sleep: By promoting relaxation and calming the nervous system, Wall Pilates can lead to deeper, more restful sleep, which is crucial for stress recovery.

Mindfulness and breath work: Focusing on your breath and present-moment awareness during exercises fosters mental clarity and reduces anxiety.

Increased endorphins: Exercise releases natural mood boosters that combat stress and elevate your mood.

Sense of accomplishment: Completing exercises, even gentle ones, builds confidence and reduces stress by fostering a sense of self-efficacy.

How Exercise Influences Stress Levels

It's no secret that exercise is good for you, but how does it influence stress levels?

Lowers cortisol levels: Cortisol is a stress hormone, and exercise helps regulate its production, leading to a calmer response to stressful situations.

Increases brain-derived neurotrophic factor (BDNF): BDNF is a protein that fosters the development and longevity of your brain cells, which can improve mood and cognitive function, both of which are crucial for stress resilience.

Reduces inflammation: Chronic stress can contribute to inflammation and is linked to various health problems. Exercise helps reduce inflammation, improving overall well-being and stress management.

Incorporating Stress-Reducing Wall Pilates into Daily Routine

The beauty of Wall Pilates lies in its adaptability. Start with 10-15 minutes daily, finding a quiet space in your home. Here are some ways you can:

Morning Wake-Up: To wake up your body and mind, do a gentle Wall Pilates exercise first thing in the morning. Focus on moving slowly and deliberately to start the day with a sense of calm.

Lunch Break: Do some Wall Pilates stretches during a short break in the middle of the day. This can help ease the stress from standing or sitting for a long time.

Before Bed Wind-Down: To wind down in the evening, do some relaxing Wall Pilates movements. This can help your body and mind prepare for a good night's sleep.

Quick Reset for a Stressful Situation: Do Wall Pilates to calm down quickly when stressed. Moving with awareness for a few minutes can help you calm down and get your mind back on track.

Include Breathing Techniques: Combine wall Pilates moves with deep breathing techniques. This can strengthen the stress-relieving effects and help you relax.

Tips for Relaxation during Wall Pilates Exercises

Focus on your breath: Deep, controlled breaths activate your parasympathetic nervous system, promoting relaxation. Use visualisation techniques to imagine your breath washing away stress with each exhale.

Gentle stretches: Hold stretches for longer, allowing your body to release tension fully. Focus on the sensations in your muscles and mindfully acknowledge any resistance.

Positive affirmations: Repeat positive statements about calmness and self-compassion as you move. Words have power; positive affirmations can shift your mindset and promote relaxation.

Music and ambience: Create a calming environment with soothing music, natural light, or aromatherapy. Surround yourself with elements that enhance your sense of peace and tranquillity.

Stress Assessment for Seniors

Before embarking on your stress-reduction journey, understanding your stressors is critical.

Health concerns: Managing chronic conditions or facing new health challenges can be overwhelming.

Loss of loved ones: Grieving the loss of spouses, friends, or family members can bring intense emotional stress.

Retirement adjustments: Adjusting to a new lifestyle post-retirement may occasionally result in isolation or a sense of purpose.

Financial worries: Concerns about bills, healthcare costs, or maintaining independence can weigh heavily.

Identifying your triggers empowers you to target them effectively with Wall Pilates practices.

Breathing Techniques for Stress Management

Breathing techniques are a cornerstone of stress management in Wall Pilates. Here are two simple yet powerful options:

4-7-8 Breathing: Inhale slowly for 4 seconds, hold for 7 seconds, and exhale completely for 8 seconds. Repeat for for 3 - 5 minutes. This rhythmic breathing calms the nervous system and promotes relaxation.

Diaphragmatic Breathing: Place one hand on your stomach and the other on your chest. As you inhale, feel your stomach expand, not your chest. Exhale slowly, drawing your belly button towards your spine. This deep breathing engages your diaphragm, promoting relaxation and reducing stress hormones.

Alternate nostril breathing: Close one nostril with your thumb and inhale slowly. Close the other nostril with your ring finger and exhale. Repeat, alternating nostrils with each breath. Continue for 5-10 minutes.

Stress Reduction Maintenance Between Wall Pilates Sessions

The benefits of Wall Pilates extend beyond your practice sessions. Here's how to maintain calm throughout the day:

Mindful Moments: Throughout the day, take short mindfulness breaks. Close your eyes, focus on your breath, and acknowledge your internal state. Practice gratitude for the present moment and let go of worries.

Movement Breaks: Engage in mindful stretching, gentle walks, or light yoga poses throughout the day to release tension and boost your mood. Even small movements can have a significant impact.

Positive Reflections: Journal about your daily experiences, identifying both challenges and joyous moments. Focus on solutions and reframe challenges with a positive lens.

Connect with Loved Ones: Social interaction fosters a sense of belonging and reduces stress. Share laughter, conversation, and activities with loved ones to boost your emotional well-being.

Nutrition and Hydration for Stress Reduction

What you eat and drink can significantly impact your stress levels. So;

Fuel your body with nutrient-rich foods: Opt for whole grains, fruits, vegetables, and lean proteins. These help to provide essential vitamins and minerals that support your nervous system and overall well-being, enhancing your stress resilience.

Limit processed foods and sugary drinks: These can contribute to inflammation and blood sugar swings, exacerbating stress symptoms. Choose healthier alternatives like water, unsweetened tea, and natural fruits for sweetness.

Stay hydrated: Dehydration can worsen stress symptoms. Drink plenty of water throughout the day to support your body's natural stress response mechanisms.

Integrating Stress Reduction with Other Forms of Exercise

Walking or swimming: Low-impact activities that improve mood and reduce stress hormones.

Gardening: Connecting with nature and engaging in physical activity is a double dose of stress relief. Immersing yourself in nature has a calming effect on the mind and body. Take a walk in a park or your backyard, breathing in the fresh air and appreciating the natural beauty around you.

Dancing: Move your body to music! Dancing is a fun and uplifting way to release stress and improve your mood. Put on your favourite tunes and let loose!

Stress Reduction Exercises for Specific Muscle Groups

Neck and Shoulders: Gentle neck rolls, shoulder shrugs, and arm circles can release tension in these areas, often holding onto stress.

Jaw: Clench and release your jaw muscles, followed by gentle side-to-side movements to alleviate jaw tension associated with stress.

Hands and Forearms: Hand stretches, finger stretches, and forearm releases can ease tension built up from daily activities and contribute to overall stress reduction.

Stress Challenges and Solutions

We all experience stress differently, but some common triggers include tight deadlines, financial worries, or even physical discomfort. Wall Pilates addresses these challenges through targeted exercises and mindfulness techniques:

Are you feeling overwhelmed? Deep breathing exercises against the wall and gentle stretches can ease tension and clear your mind.

Are you struggling with sleeplessness? Relaxing poses like a wall child's pose (*Chapter four*) promote relaxation and prepare your body for restful sleep.

Are you experiencing physical pain? Gentle mobility exercises tailored to your specific issues can improve flexibility and reduce discomfort, contributing to overall stress reduction.

Wall Pilates for Emotional Well-being

Beyond physical benefits, Wall Pilates fosters emotional well-being by:

Boosting mood: Combining physical activity and mindfulness releases endorphins, natural mood-elevating chemicals.

Reducing stress hormones: Regular practice of Wall Pilates can lower cortisol levels, the stress hormone, leading to a calmer emotional state.

Promoting self-compassion: The gentle nature of Wall Pilates encourages self-care and acceptance, fostering a positive relationship with your body and mind.

***

Preview of Exercise List

B ELOW IS A LIST of stress reduction wall pilates exercises with different adaptation levels. Practice makes perfect, and stress reduction is not a race. Explore the exercises using the wall as your trusty friend.

Exercise List

Beginner

Warm-Up (two minutes):

Gentle Neck Rolls: Gently roll your head clockwise and counter-clockwise, feeling the stretch in your neck muscles. Repeat five times in each direction.

Arm Circles: With your arms out at shoulder height, move your arms forward and backward, making small circles, gradually increasing their size. Repeat ten times in each direction.

Wall Mindful Breathing (two minutes):

Sit comfortably with your back on the wall. Place your hands gently on your belly. Close your eyes if comfortable, or gaze downward softly.

Breathe deeply and slowly through your nose, feeling your belly rise and fall with each inhale and exhale. Focus on the present moment and let go of thoughts or worries. Imagine breathing in calmness and exhaling tension.

Wall Meditation Pose (two minutes):

Stand back against a wall with your feet hip-width apart and about an inch away from the wall. Lean your back gently against the wall, keeping your spine straight.

Close your eyes if comfortable, or softly gaze downward. Focus on your breath and the feeling of your body against the wall. Observe any thoughts or sensations without judgment.

Wall Body Scan Meditation (two minutes):

Lie on your back on the floor with your legs extended and feet against the wall. Close your eyes and focus on your breath.

Slowly bring your attention to different body parts, starting with your toes and moving upwards. Notice any sensations, tightness, or relaxation in each area. Observe without judgment and let go of any tension.

Wall Pilates Flow Sequence (four minutes):

This sequence includes gentle Pilates exercises using the wall for support.

Cat-Cow (two minutes): Start on all fours with your hands and knees on the floor, hip-width apart. Inhale as you arch your back and look up like a cow; exhale as you round your back and tuck your chin to your chest. Repeat 5-10 times.

Leg Slides (two minutes): Sit on the floor with your back against the wall and your legs extended. Slowly slide one heel towards the wall, keeping your leg straight. Slide it back and repeat with the other leg. Repeat 5-10 times on each side.

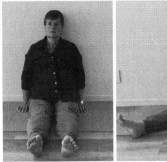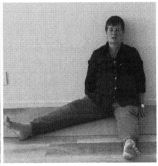

Cool-Down (two minutes):

Deep Breathing: Repeat the mindful breathing exercise from the warm-up.

Quad stretch: Hold onto the wall for support and bring your heel towards your buttocks. Repeat on both sides for 30 seconds.

Intermediate

Warm-Up (two minutes): Same as beginner.

Wall Pilates with Soft Music (four minutes):

Perform the Wall Pilates Flow Sequence from the beginner level while listening to calming music. Focus on the flow of movement and the connection between your breath and body.

Wall Visualisation Exercise (five minutes):

Stand with your back against the wall with your eyes closed. Imagine yourself in a peaceful place, feeling calm and relaxed.

Focus on the sensations and emotions associated with the place. Feel the stress melt away as you immerse yourself in your visualisation.

Cool-Down (two minutes): Same as beginner.

Advanced

Warm-Up (two minutes): Same as beginner.

Wall Mindful Walking (three minutes):

Stand with your side next to the wall, your feet hip-width apart, about an inch away. Close your eyes (optional) and take slow, deep breaths.

Focus your attention on the feeling of your feet on the ground and the sensations in your body with each step. Slowly lift one foot a few inches off the ground and gently place it back down in front of the other foot, focusing on the movement and sound.

Repeat with the other foot, continuing your mindful walking meditation for three minutes back and forth.

Wall Relaxation Pose (three minutes):

Stand back against the wall with your hips about an inch away. Slowly slide down the wall until your back is fully supported, knees bent, and feet flat on the floor as if you are sitting.

Extend your arms overhead or let them hang naturally at your sides. Close your eyes and focus on your breath, taking slow, deep inhales and exhales.

Let your body completely relax against the wall, releasing tension. Visualise yourself sinking deeper into relaxation with each breath. Stay in this pose for three minutes or as long as comfortable.

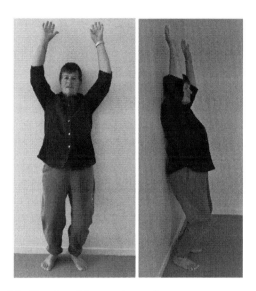

Wall Gratitude Meditation (three minutes):

Stand back against the wall with your feet hip-width apart and arms at your sides. Close your eyes (optional) and take a few deep breaths to centre yourself. Bring to mind something you're grateful for, big or small.

Visualise placing this gratitude on the wall behind you, like a warm light or symbol. Continue reflecting on and placing more things you're grateful for, building a wall of gratitude behind you.

Feel the warmth and appreciation spreading through your body. Stay mindful for three minutes or as long as you are comfortable.

Cool-Down (two minutes): Same as beginner.

Now, use these exercises to relieve the weight of stress on your shoulders. They are sure to leave you revitalised and happy. In the next chapter, we will see how exactly wall pilates can help you get better sleep.

CHAPTER 10

WALL PILATES FOR BETTER SLEEP

"Sleep is the golden chain that ties health and our bodies together."

Are you tossing and turning throughout the night? Do you want a good night's sleep but are overwhelmed by the number of sleep aids and treatments available? Sleep issues happen at any age but can be particularly challenging for seniors. Allow Wall Pilates to assist you with more restful evenings and fresh vitality. Reclaim your nights and enjoy waking up feeling rejuvenated. Wall Pilates enables you to naturally increase your sleep quality, enhancing overall health and quality of life.

Understanding Sleep and Aging

As we age, our sleep patterns change. We may experience shorter sleep durations, lighter sleep, and more frequent awakenings, which can be attributed to various factors, including hormonal changes, medical conditions, and lifestyle habits. However, it's important to remember that quality sleep remains crucial for seniors' well-being.

Importance of Quality Sleep for Seniors

Adequate sleep is essential for preserving cognitive function, physical health, and emotional well-being as seniors. It influences everything from memory and focus to immune function and mood management. Poor sleep can raise the risk of chronic illnesses such as diabetes, depression and heart disease.

How Wall Pilates Contributes to Better Sleep

Wall Pilates doesn't just address the physical aspects of sleep; it tackles the root causes of sleeplessness. Here's how:

Stress Reduction: Gentle exercises and mindful movements release tension and anxiety, promoting relaxation and preparing your body for sleep.

Improved Flexibility and Mobility: Tight muscles and joint stiffness can disrupt sleep. Wall Pilates stretches, and exercises enhance flexibility and mobility, easing discomfort and promoting peaceful rest.

Better Body Awareness and Relaxation: Focusing on mindful movements and breathing techniques cultivate body awareness and deep relaxation, quieting and preparing the mind for sleep.

Reduced Pain and Discomfort: Many seniors experience chronic pain that disrupts sleep. Wall Pilates exercises can address specific pain points, improve posture, and promote overall comfort, leading to better sleep quality.

Sleep Hygiene Tips for Seniors

Creating healthy sleep habits, also known as sleep hygiene, is crucial for improving sleep quality at any age. Here are some critical tips for seniors:

Stick to a steady sleep routine: Aim to go to sleep and wake up at consistent times every day, including weekends. This will help regulate your body's innate sleep-wake rhythm.

Create a relaxing bedtime routine: Before bed, read a book, listen to music, or take a warm bath. Avoid activities like watching TV or using electronic devices, as this can stimulate the brain.

Optimise your sleep environment: Make sure your bedroom is dark, quiet, and cool. Use comfortable bedding and invest in blackout curtains if necessary.

Limit caffeine and alcohol: Avoid caffeine in the afternoon and evening, as it has the potential to interfere with sleep. Limit alcohol intake, as this can disrupt sleep patterns.

Engage in regular exercise: Regular physical activity can improve sleep quality, but avoid strenuous exercise close to bedtime.

Tips for Relaxation and Mindfulness Before Bed

Developing a pre-sleep ritual that promotes relaxation and mindfulness can significantly improve sleep quality. Here are some suggestions:

Deep breathing exercises: Lie comfortably and focus on slow, deep breaths from your diaphragm. Breathe in for a count of four, hold for a count of four, and exhale for a count of eight. Repeat for several minutes.

Progressive muscle relaxation: Alternate between tensing and relaxing various muscle groups in your body, beginning from your toes and progressing upward. This technique can aid in alleviating tension and encouraging relaxation.

Sleep Assessment for Seniors

It is essential to look at your sleep patterns and habits to stay healthy and happy, especially as we become seniors. Here's an easy way for seniors to check how well they sleep:

Sleep Duration: Track the number of hours you sleep each night. Most seniors need between 7 and 9 hours of sleep each night to be healthy.

Sleep Quality: Rate your sleep quality on a scale of 1 to 10, with 10 being the best. Think about how long it takes to fall asleep, how often you wake up at night, and how rested you feel in the morning.

Sleep Environment: Evaluate your sleep environment. Make sure your bedroom is dark and quiet and has the right temperature. If necessary, you could use earplugs, an eye mask, or a white noise machine.

Bedtime Routine: Assess your bedtime routine. Set up a relaxing routine before bed to let your body know it's time to be tired. Some examples of this are reading, taking a warm bath, or listening to music that makes you feel better.

Daily Habits: Consider your daily habits that may affect your sleep. Don't drink coffee, smoke, or eat big meals right before bed. Aim to work out regularly, but don't do anything too intense right before bed.

Medical Conditions: Take note of any medical conditions that may affect your sleep, for example, sleep apnea, restless legs syndrome, or chronic pain. Talk to your healthcare provider about how to handle things properly.

Medications: Go over any medications you're taking. Some medicines have been proven to make it harder to sleep.

Nutrition and Hydration for Better Sleep

The beverages and food you consume can have a significant impact on the quality of your sleep. Here are some strategies to help:

Avoid heavy meals before bed: A light, healthy dinner 3-4 hours before sleep promotes digestion and prevents sleep disturbances.

Stay hydrated: Dehydration can disrupt sleep. Drink plenty of water throughout the day and avoid diuretics like coffee and alcohol before bedtime.

Incorporate sleep-promoting foods: Foods rich in magnesium, tryptophan, and melatonin can support restful sleep. Consider cherries, bananas, almonds, and yogurt.

Sleep-Inducing Exercises for Specific Muscles

Specific muscle groups hold tension that can disrupt sleep. Wall Pilates offers targeted exercises for relaxation:

Neck and shoulders: Wall neck stretches (*Chapter two*), gentle shoulder rolls (*Chapter two*), and supported wall child's pose (*Chapter four*) can release tension in these areas.

Back: Wall cat-cow poses (*Chapter two*) and wall angels (*Chapter eight*) can improve flexibility and promote relaxation in your back muscles.

Legs and feet: Wall calf stretches(*Chapter one*), wall hamstring stretches (*Chapter one*), and gentle foot rotations can ease tension and improve circulation in your lower extremities.

Sleep Challenges and Solutions

We all experience sleep challenges differently, but some common culprits include:

Racing thoughts: Calming stretches like wall hamstring stretches and supported wall savasana promote relaxation and quiet the mind.

Tight muscles: Gentle mobility exercises like seated wall spinal twists and wall hip flexor stretches (*See both exercises below*) release tension, preparing your body for sleep.

Irregular sleep schedule: Sticking to a consistent sleep routine is crucial. Wall Pilates can be incorporated into your evening wind-down to signal to your body that it's time to prepare for sleep.

Wall Pilates for Evening Routines

Establishing a calming bedtime ritual can significantly enhance the quality of your sleep. Wall Pilates offers a perfect addition to your evenings:

Start with gentle stretches: Prepare your body for relaxation with wall hamstring stretches (*Chapter One*).

Focus on deep breathing: Techniques like wall diaphragmatic breathing and alternate nostril breathing (*Chapter Nine*) promote relaxation and calm the nervous system.

End with supported poses: Wind down with calming poses like the supported wall child's pose (*Chapter Four*) to ease into sleep.

Sleep-Inducing Breathing Techniques

You should know that your breath plays a crucial role in sleep quality. Wall Pilates incorporates deep breathing exercises like diaphragmatic breathing and alternate nostril breathing (*As shown in chapter nine*).

These techniques help activate the parasympathetic nervous system, which promotes relaxation and helps prepare the body for restful sleep.

***

Preview of Exercise List

Now, LET'S MOVE ON to the exciting world of Wall Pilates to help you sleep better. Each exercise has thorough instructions, modifications, and progressions to make it fit your needs and preferences. Start your journey one gentle step at a time to sleep well at night and feel refreshed in the morning!

Exercise List

Beginner

Warm-Up (two minutes):

Arm Circles: With your arms stretched out at shoulder height, make small circles with your arms forward and backward, increasing the size of the circles slowly. Repeat ten times in each direction for one minute.

Deep Breathing: Sit or stand comfortably and take slow, deep breaths through your nose and out your mouth. Focus on feeling your belly rise and fall with each breath. Repeat for five breaths.

Wall Child's Pose (two minutes):

Kneel on the floor with your toes together and sit back on your heels. Extend your arms forward, resting your palms on the wall. Rest your forehead on the floor, with your chest close to your thighs.

Walk your hands out slightly if needed for comfort. Relax your shoulders and breathe deeply. Hold for as long as desired.

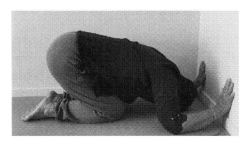

Wall Legs Up the Wall Pose (two minutes):

Lie on your back on the floor with your legs extended. Slide your legs up the wall until your body forms an L shape. Relax your arms at your sides or rest them on your belly.

Breathe deeply and slowly, feeling the heaviness of your legs and the relaxation in your lower back. Stay in this pose for two minutes.

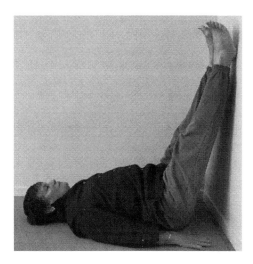

Wall Spinal Twist (ten repetitions on each side):

Sit on the floor facing the wall with your knees bent and feet flat on the floor. Place your right hand on the wall in front of you and your left hand on your right knee.

Gently twist your torso to the left, looking over your left shoulder. Hold for four seconds, then inhale as you return to the centre. Repeat ten times on each side.

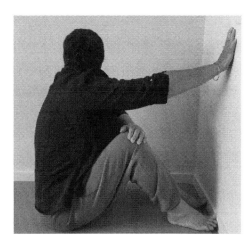

Cool-Down (two minutes):

Deep Breathing: Repeat the mindful breathing exercise from the warm-up.

Chest stretch: Clasp your hands behind your back and gently open your chest, pushing your shoulders back.

Intermediate

Warm-Up (two minutes): Same as beginner.

Wall Relaxation Pose (four minutes):

Stand with your back against the wall with your hips about an inch away. Slowly slide down the wall until your back is fully supported, knees bent, and feet flat on the floor.

Extend your arms overhead, resting them on the wall or letting them hang naturally at your sides. Close your eyes and focus on your breath, taking slow, deep inhales and exhales.

Let your body completely relax against the wall, releasing tension. Visualise yourself sinking deeper into relaxation with each breath. Stay in this pose for four minutes or as long as comfortable.

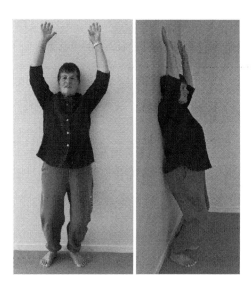

Wall Deep Breathing (three minutes):

Sit on the floor with your back against the wall and your legs extended. Place one hand on your belly and the other on your chest.

Breathe deeply through your nose, feeling your belly expand with each inhale. Exhale slowly through your mouth, feeling your belly contract and chest sink.

Focus on the rhythm of your breath and let go of any thoughts or worries. Continue deep breathing for three minutes.

Wall Forward Bend (three repetitions):

Stand facing a wall with your feet hip-width apart and your toes a few inches away from the base of the wall. Slowly lean forward and place your hands flat on the wall.

Walk your hands down the wall as far as comfortable, keeping your back straight. Stop when you feel a gentle stretch in your shoulders, back, and hamstrings.

Relax your neck and shoulders as you hold the stretch for 15-30 seconds, breathing deeply. Slowly walk your hands back up the wall and return to the starting position.

You can repeat the wall forward bend three times, gradually increasing the stretch as your flexibility improves.

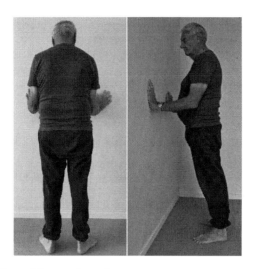

Wall Shoulder Stand (one minute):

Lie on your back on the floor with your legs extended up the wall. Press your hips and lower back into the floor for support.

Lift your legs straight up towards the ceiling, keeping them together. Breathe deeply and hold for one minute seconds, or as long as possible.

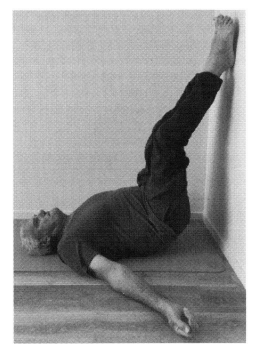

Cool-Down (two minutes): Same as beginner.

Advanced

Warm-Up (two minutes): Same as beginner.

Wall Abdominal Breathing (five minutes):

Lie on your back on the floor with your legs extended and feet against the wall.

Place one hand on your belly and the other on your chest. Breathe deeply through your nose, focusing on expanding your belly outwards, not your chest.

Exhale slowly through your mouth, drawing your belly button towards your spine. Pay attention to the rise and fall of your belly with each breath, practising mindful breathing for five minutes.

Wall Hip Flexor Stretch (30 seconds on each side):

Place a pad or towel on the floor a couple of feet away from a wall. Place your right knee down on the pad and your left foot out in front of you towards the wall, knee bent and foot flat on the ground.

Rest your left hand on the wall. With your right hand, reach back and grab your right foot, lifting it. Now lean forward with your hand on the wall.

Lean forward as far as you can, hold for 30 seconds. Repeat with your other left knee on the pad.

Wall Meditation Pose (five minutes):

Stand with your back against the wall, feet flat on the floor, and knees bent at a 90-degree angle. As if sitting on an imaginary chair.

Close your eyes (optional) and take slow, deep breaths. Focus on the feeling of your body against the wall and your breath. Observe any thoughts or sensations without judgment, simply letting them come and go. Practice mindfulness and relaxation for five minutes.

Cool-Down (two minutes): Same as beginner.

Stop tossing and turning and welcome a much-needed goodnight sleep into your life. We'll meet in the next chapter, where we tackle one of the most challenging and frustrating issues many seniors face—joint mobility.

CHAPTER 11

WALL PILATES FOR JOINT MOBILITY

"Take care of your joints, and they'll take care of you."

Do stiff joints impede your regular activities and make you feel restricted? Have you convinced yourself that decreased mobility is a natural aspect of aging? I have a treat for you. If daily activities now feel like an obstacle course due to stiff joints, don't despair. While age-related changes can affect joint health, it's not inevitable; you may reclaim your agility and live a life full of movement. Wall Pilates enables you to naturally enhance joint mobility, resulting in pain-free movement throughout your body.

The Importance of Joint Mobility for Seniors

Maintaining good joint mobility is crucial for seniors as it impacts daily life. Here's why:

Improved daily activities: Enhanced flexibility allows you to efficiently perform tasks like reaching, bending, and climbing stairs.

Reduced risk of falls: Increased range of motion improves balance and coordination, making you less prone to falls and injuries.

Pain management: Gentle stretches and exercises can help reduce stiffness and pain, which can be associated with arthritis and other joint conditions.

How Aging Affects Joint Health

Several age-related changes can affect joint health:

Cartilage breakdown: Cartilage, the cushioning material in your joints, naturally wears down with age, leading to stiffness and pain.

Muscle loss: Loss of muscle mass reduces strength and stability, further impacting joint health and flexibility.

Decreased bone density: Osteoporosis can weaken bones and increase the risk of fractures, impacting joint mobility.

Decreased flexibility: Connective tissues like tendons and ligaments become less elastic with age, restricting joint movement.

Benefits of Wall Pilates for Joint Mobility

Wall Pilates offers a unique approach to address these age-related changes and improve joint mobility:

Gentle exercises: Wall-based exercises provide support and minimise stress on joints, making them safe and effective for all fitness levels.

Targeted stretches: concentrate on enhancing flexibility in the knees, hips, and shoulders.

Muscle strengthening: Exercises engage various muscle groups, improving stability and supporting joint movement.

Mindful movement: Focusing on proper alignment and movement patterns enhances coordination and body awareness, reducing the risk of injury.

Incorporating Joint Mobility Exercises into Daily Routine

While Wall Pilates offers structured activities, incorporating simple joint mobility exercises throughout your day can further improve your joint mobility:

Morning Stretch Routine: To wake up your body, start your day with light joint movement exercises, like shoulder rolls, hip circles, and knee lifts.

While Watching TV: Perform ankle circles, wrist circles, and neck stretches during commercial breaks or between episodes.

At the Office: Take short breaks to stand up and stretch your wrists, fingers, and shoulders to prevent stiffness from prolonged sitting.

During Phone Calls: Use phone calls as an opportunity to stand up and perform calf raises and neck stretches while chatting.

Cooking or Waiting for Food: While preparing food to cook or heat up, perform standing leg swings, side bends, and arm circles to keep your joints mobile.

Walking: Incorporate joint-friendly movements like knee lifts, ankle circles, and arm swings into your daily dog walks or when walking if you don't have a dog.

Wall Pilates for Enhanced Range of Motion

Our joints rely on a healthy range of motion to function correctly. Wall Pilates addresses this by incorporating targeted exercises and stretches specifically designed to improve flexibility and movement in your:

Spine: Gentle twists and cat-cow poses against the wall (*Chapter two*) help increase spinal mobility, promoting good posture and overall functional movement.

Shoulders: Wall arm circles and modified shoulder stretches enhance the mobility of your shoulder joints, reducing tightness and discomfort.

Hips: Side leg lifts (*Chapter five*) against the wall improve hip mobility and flexibility, promoting pain-free movement and balance.

Knees and ankles: Gentle wall stretches and supported wall squats (*Chapter one*) target the knee and ankle joints, increasing flexibility and reducing stiffness.

Remember, this is just a glimpse into the vast array of exercises Wall Pilates offers for improved joint mobility. More detailed exercises and modifications are included below in the exercise lists.

Tips for Maintaining Joint Mobility during Exercises

Maintaining proper form during your Wall Pilates exercises is crucial to ensure joint safety and maximise benefits. Here are some essential tips:

Maintain a neutral spine throughout the exercises. Avoid slouching or arching your back.

Activate your core muscles for stability and support. This protects your lower back and prevents unnecessary stress on your joints.

Breathe profoundly and rhythmically throughout the movements. This helps to improve circulation and oxygen delivery to your joints, promoting healing and mobility.

Joint Mobility Assessment for Seniors

As we age, assessing our joint mobility becomes crucial for identifying potential limitations and preventing injuries. Below are a few straightforward assessments you can conduct at home:

Shoulder range of motion: Reach your arms overhead and behind your back to assess your shoulder mobility.

Hip range of motion: Sit on the floor and try to reach your toes with your hands, keeping your back straight.

Spine flexibility: Lie on your back and hug your knees to your chest, then try to touch your forehead to your knees.

Knowing areas of stiffness can help you tailor your exercises and know which parts of your body need more priority. If you experience pain or difficulty performing these movements, consulting a healthcare professional is recommended to discuss personalised exercises and strategies to improve your joint mobility safely.

Wall Pilates for Arthritis Relief and Joint Health

Pilates exercises against a wall can offer significant benefits for individuals coping with arthritis. These gentle routines alleviate discomfort, enhance mobility, and bolster the muscles surrounding your joints, thereby improving joint health and function.

Joint Mobility Maintenance Between Wall Pilates Sessions

While Wall Pilates offers incredible benefits, maintaining joint mobility requires consistency and goes beyond your practice sessions. Here are some tips for ongoing joint health:

Movement throughout the day: Break up long periods of sitting with gentle stretches, walks, or simple movements like ankle circles.

Self-myofascial release: Use foam rollers or massage balls to release muscle tension and trigger points, improving joint mobility.

Staying active: Engage in activities you enjoy, like walking, swimming, or dancing. This keeps your joints moving and helps maintain flexibility.

Nutrition and Hydration for Optimal Joint Health

Nourishing your body with the proper nutrients is crucial for joint health. Here's what to keep in mind:

Stay hydrated: Drinking sufficient water helps lubricate your joints and promotes overall flexibility.

Choose anti-inflammatory foods: Include fruits, vegetables, and whole grains rich in antioxidants, which can help combat inflammation and reduce discomfort.

Incorporate healthy fats: Omega-3 fatty acids in fatty fish, nuts, and seeds can contribute to joint health and reduce inflammation.

Joint Mobility Challenges and Solutions

Everyone experiences different joint mobility challenges, but some common concerns include:

Stiffness and pain: Wall Pilates offers targeted stretches and gentle exercises to address specific areas of tightness and discomfort, promoting increased flexibility and reducing pain.

Limited range of motion: Specific exercises targeting individual joints gradually increase your range of motion, allowing for more fluid and unrestricted movement.

Loss of balance and coordination: Wall exercises provide support and stability while practising balance and coordination exercises, improving your confidence and safety as you move.

Injury recovery: Wall Pilates exercises can support rehabilitation and injury recovery by promoting blood flow and gentle strengthening.

Wall Pilates for Joint Stability

While improving flexibility is crucial, joint stability is essential for pain-free movement and injury prevention. Wall Pilates incorporates exercises that target the muscles surrounding your joints, strengthening them to provide support and stability. Examples include:

Wall squats: Performed with your back against the wall, these squats engage your leg muscles, strengthening the hips and knees, which is crucial for maintaining lower body stability.

Wall arm circles: These gentle circles, with variations in arm position, activate the shoulder muscles, promoting stability and improved range of motion.

Side-lying leg lifts against the wall: Performed on your side with one leg resting against the wall for support, this exercise strengthens the hip abductors, which is crucial for maintaining hip stability and preventing pain.

Joint-Friendly Breathing Techniques

Proper breathing plays a vital role in joint health. Deep breathing can help you relax and get more blood flowing to your joints, making them less stiff and more mobile. For this method, you inhale deeply through your nose until you feel your belly expand, and then slowly let out your breath through pursed lips.

You can add more breathing techniques to your exercise, such as alternate nostril breathing, which is when you breathe in through one nostril and out through the other. This can help you relax and move your joints more easily.

***

Preview of Exercise List in This Chapter

B ELOW IS A FRIENDLY exercise list for seniors at all levels. Regularly practising Wall Pilates exercises and incorporating these techniques can significantly improve joint mobility and overall well-being. Start your journey towards pain-free movement and rediscover the joy of movement.

Exercise List

Beginner:

Warm-Up (two minutes):

Gentle Neck Rolls: Gently roll your head clockwise and counter-clockwise, feeling the stretch in your neck muscles. Repeat five times in each direction for a minute.

Arm Circles: With your arms outstretched at shoulder height, move your arms forward and backward, making small circles. Slowly increase the size of the circles. Repeat five times in each direction for a minute.

Wall Hip Circles (ten repetitions in each direction):

Stand with your back against the wall with your feet hip-width apart and about an inch away from the wall. Place your hands on your hips.

Gently make small circles with your hips, feeling the movement in your lower back and glutes. Focus on keeping your core activated and your back straight throughout the exercise. Repeat ten circles in each direction.

Wall Ankle Circles (ten repetitions in each direction):

Stand facing the wall with your feet hip-width apart and about an inch away from the wall. Hold onto the wall for support.

Make small circles with your foot, rotating your ankles clockwise and counter-clockwise. Focus on using your ankle muscles to move your foot, not your leg.

Do ten circles in each direction, move to the next foot and repeat.

Wall Knee Flexion and Extension (ten repetitions):

Stand with the wall on your side, your feet hip-width apart and about an inch away from the wall. Hold onto the wall for support.

Slowly lift one knee towards your chest, keeping your other leg straight. Hold for ten seconds, then slowly lower your leg. Repeat ten times on each leg.

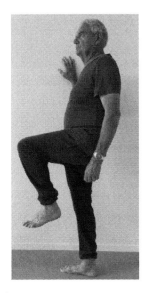

Cool-Down (two minutes):

Deep Breathing: Sit or stand comfortably and take slow, deep breaths through your nose and out your mouth for one minute.

Quad stretch: Hold onto the wall for support and bring your heel towards your buttocks. Do this for a minute, alternating legs.

Intermediate:

Warm-Up (two minutes): Same as beginner.

Wall Shoulder Rolls (ten repetitions in each direction):

Stand facing the wall with your feet hip-width apart. Raise one arm out to the sides at shoulder height and raise the other forward, resting your palm on the wall.

Make small circles with one shoulder (extended arm at the side), forward and backward. Focus on keeping your shoulders relaxed and your core engaged. Do ten circles in each direction, switching hand positions after one minute.

Wall Wrist Flexor Stretch (two minutes):

Stand facing the wall with your feet hip-width apart and about an inch away from the wall. Place your hands flat on the wall at shoulder height, fingers pointing upwards.

Lean forward gently, keeping your back straight and core engaged. Feel the stretch in your forearms and wrists.

Hold for 20 - 30 seconds, lean back up, and repeat for two minutes.

Wall Neck Tilts (ten repetitions on each side):

Stand with your back against the wall with your feet hip-width apart and about an inch away from the wall. Tilt your head to one side, bringing your ear towards your shoulder.

Hold for 3 - 5 seconds, then slowly return to the centre. Repeat ten times on each side.

Cool-Down (two minutes): Same as beginner.

Advanced:

Warm-Up (two minutes): Same as beginner.

Wall Elbow Circles (ten repetitions each):

Stand with the wall to your side, your feet hip-width apart. Put your left hand on your shoulder and your right hand on the wall. Your elbow should be at shoulder level and pointing out.

Make a circle with your elbow. Breathe out as you start and breathe in when you finish the rotation. Focus on keeping your shoulders relaxed and your core engaged. Switch hand positions and repeat ten circles for each elbow.

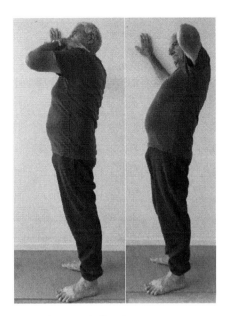

Wall Toe Taps (ten repetitions each foot):

Stand facing the wall with your feet hip-width apart and hands on the wall for support. Gently tap one foot up and down against the wall, keeping your heel on the floor and your leg straight.

Focus on using your ankle muscles to control the movement. Repeat ten times on each foot.

Wall Spinal Twist (ten repetitions on each side):

Stand with your back to the wall with your feet hip-width apart and about an inch away from the wall. Place your hands on your shoulders, elbows out to the sides.

Gently twist your torso to one side, looking over your shoulder. Focus on keeping your hips facing forward, your core engaged, and your back straight.

Hold for five seconds, then return to the centre and repeat on the other side. Repeat ten times on each side.

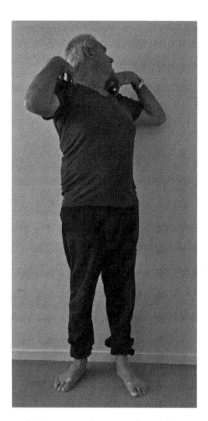

Wall Quadriceps Stretch (30 seconds on each side):

Stand facing the wall with your feet hip-width apart and one hand holding the wall for support.

Lift one foot off the ground, bending it at the knee. Grab the top of your foot or ankle with your hand and gently pull it towards your buttocks, feeling the stretch in the front of your thigh.

Keep your other leg straight and your core engaged. Hold for 30 seconds on each side.

Wall Cat-Cow (ten repetitions):

Kneel facing the wall, hands and knees on the floor, hip-width apart. As you inhale, round your back, tucking your chin to your chest like a cat. As you exhale, arch your back, looking up towards the ceiling like a cow.

Focus on keeping your hands and knees in the same position throughout the movement and engaging your core muscles. Repeat ten repetitions.

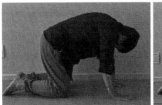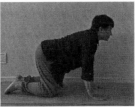

Cool-Down (two minutes): Same as beginner.

Now, you can go ahead and resume your regular activities or activities you sadly had to drop because of the restrictions in your joints. Reclaim your agility and a daily life full of movement. The next chapter shows how Wall Pilates helps with cardiovascular health, and it is one you would want to take advantage of. See you in the next chapter.

CHAPTER 12

WALL PILATES FOR CARDIOVASCULAR HEALTH

"The best way to keep your heart in shape is to keep moving."

Have you been told that strengthening your heart requires strenuous gym sessions? Are you feeling sluggish and out of breath? Are you aware that your heart health could improve with some improvement and a boost, but you need to figure out what to do and where to start? Allow wall pilates to help you, then. Discover how gentle exercises, targeted movements, and mindful breathing can improve cardiovascular health, regardless of age or fitness level.

Understanding Cardiovascular Health in Seniors

A healthy heart ensures that blood flows properly through your body, giving your brain, muscles, lungs, and other systems oxygen and nutrients. Our cardiovascular system, including the heart, blood vessels, and blood, has changed naturally as we age and become seniors.

These changes are regular, and keeping your heart healthy is essential for general health. Heart disease is the top cause of death in the world. Things that raise your risk include high blood pressure, high cholesterol, and not being active enough.

Benefits of Cardiovascular Exercise for Aging Adults

Engaging in regular physical activity offers numerous benefits, even low-impact exercises, for cardiovascular health in seniors:

Improves heart function: Exercise strengthens the heart muscle, allowing it to pump blood more efficiently throughout the body, delivering oxygen and nutrients to vital organs.

Low blood pressure: Consistent physical activity can efficiently reduce blood pressure, thereby decreasing the likelihood of heart disease and stroke.

Boosts circulation: Exercise improves blood flow, delivering oxygen and nutrients to tissues more effectively and eliminating waste products.

Increases energy levels: Regular physical activity promotes better sleep and enhances overall stamina, energising you throughout the day.

How Wall Pilates Contributes to Cardiovascular Health

While Wall Pilates may not be a high-intensity workout, it offers unique benefits for cardiovascular health for us seniors:

Low-impact movements: Wall Pilates exercises are gentle on the joints, making them suitable for individuals with restrictions or beginners to exercise.

Increased heart rate: While not as intense as running or swimming, some Wall Pilates exercises can elevate your heart rate, promoting cardiovascular benefits.

Improved circulation: The fluid motions of Wall Pilates aid in enhancing blood circulation throughout the body, supporting overall cardiovascular well-being.

Enhanced lung capacity: Deep, mindful breathing exercises incorporated into Wall Pilates practice can improve lung function, aiding overall cardiovascular health.

Incorporating Cardiovascular Wall Pilates into Daily Routine

Achieving the advantages of Wall Pilates for heart health relies on consistency. Aim for at least 30 minutes of moderate-intensity exercise on most days of the week, which you can divide into shorter, more manageable sessions throughout the day. Here are some suggestions for integrating Wall Pilates into your everyday schedule:

Start with short sessions: Begin with 10-15 minute sessions and gradually increase the duration as your fitness level improves.

Find a time that works for you: Whether morning, afternoon, or evening, choose a time that fits your schedule and stick to it.

Make it a routine: Schedule your Wall Pilates sessions in your calendar like any other appointment.

Listen to your body: Don't push yourself too hard, especially if you're new to exercise. Take breaks when needed and gradually increase the intensity.

Tips for Maintaining Cardiovascular Health during Exercises

Here are some additional tips to ensure safe and effective cardiovascular training with Wall Pilates:

Stay hydrated: Drink plenty of water before, during, and after your practice to stay hydrated and support your cardiovascular system.

Warm-up and cool-down: Always begin with gentle stretches and light exercises to warm up your body, and end your practice with cool-down stretches to promote recovery.

Focus on proper breathing: Deep, diaphragmatic breathing ensures proper oxygen delivery to your muscles, maximising the benefits of your exercises.

Cardiovascular Health Assessment for Seniors

While Wall Pilates offers a safe and accessible approach to improving cardiovascular health for various individuals, it's crucial to consider specific factors for seniors, so you know what's going on in your body.

Know Your Numbers: Monitor your blood pressure, cholesterol, and blood sugar levels regularly. These numbers can provide valuable insights into your cardiovascular health.

Assess Your Lifestyle: Evaluate your lifestyle habits, including diet, exercise, smoking, and alcohol consumption. Making healthy choices can significantly impact your cardiovascular health.

Check Your Heart Rate: Monitor your resting heart rate and assess how it changes during physical activity. A lower resting heart rate is generally a sign of good cardiovascular fitness.

Evaluate Your Activity Level: Assess your daily physical activity. Health experts recommend at least 150 minutes of moderate-intensity aerobic activity per week.

Assess Your Diet: Evaluate your diet and ensure it includes plenty of fruits, vegetables, whole grains, and lean proteins. Limiting saturated fats, trans fats, and sodium can also improve cardiovascular health.

Consider Your Stress Levels: Evaluate your stress levels and how they impact your cardiovascular health. Finding healthy ways to manage stress, such as meditation or wall pilates, can be beneficial.

Assess Your Weight: Check your body mass index (BMI) to assess if you are at a healthy weight. Excess weight can strain your cardiovascular system and increase your risk of heart disease.

Assess Your Family History: Consider your family history of cardiovascular disease. A family history of heart disease can increase your risk, so taking preventive measures is essential.

Cardiovascular Health Maintenance Between Wall Pilates Sessions

While Wall Pilates offers numerous benefits, it's essential to maintain healthy habits throughout the day to optimise your cardiovascular health:

Regular physical activity: Aim for at least 150 minutes of moderate or 75 minutes of vigorous-intensity exercise per week. This can include brisk walking, swimming, cycling, or other forms of exercise you enjoy.

Healthy diet: Choose a balanced diet rich in fruits, vegetables, whole grains, and lean protein. Limit saturated and trans fats, processed foods, and added sugars.

Maintaining a healthy weight: Obesity is a risk factor for cardiovascular disease. If you're overweight or obese, consult your healthcare professional for personalised guidance on weight management.

Managing stress: Chronic stress can contribute to heart problems. Practice stress-reduction techniques like meditation, yoga, or deep breathing exercises, which Wall Pilates can also support.

Nutrition and Hydration for Optimal Cardiovascular Health

What you eat and drink is vital in supporting your heart health. Here's what to focus on:

Choose heart-healthy fats: Opt for sources like olive oil, avocado, and fatty fish, which are rich in omega-3 fatty acids and benefit heart health.

Limit unhealthy fats: Minimise saturated and trans fats in processed meats, fried foods, and baked goods.

Stay hydrated: Drinking plenty of water throughout the day is crucial for optimal heart function and overall health.

Adapting Cardiovascular Exercises for Seniors with Medical Conditions

The beauty of Wall Pilates lies in its adaptability. Seniors and individuals with specific medical conditions can benefit significantly from this practice, even with modifications.

Low-impact modifications: Activities like high knees or jumping jacks (*both in Chapter five*) can be replaced with modified versions like wall marches (*Chapter five*) or wall toe taps (*Chapter seven*).

Focus on controlled movements: Maintaining proper form and controlled movements throughout exercises ensures safety and effectiveness, even at a slower pace.

Cardiovascular Challenges and Solutions

Everyone encounters challenges related to cardiovascular health. Some common ones include:

High blood pressure: Wall Pilates promotes relaxation and stress reduction, which can positively impact blood pressure levels.

High cholesterol: While exercise alone cannot directly lower cholesterol, improving cardiovascular health and maintaining a healthy weight can contribute to cholesterol management.

Low energy levels: The increased blood flow and improved oxygen circulation associated with Wall Pilates can increase energy levels throughout the day.

Wall Pilates for Improved Blood Pressure

High blood pressure, a significant risk factor for heart disease, can be positively impacted by Wall Pilates. Studies suggest that regular practice can:

Lower systolic and diastolic blood pressure: The gentle yet continuous movement and mindful breathing can activate the parasympathetic nervous system, reducing stress and lowering blood pressure.

Improve blood vessel flexibility: Gentle stretches and exercises can improve the elasticity of blood vessels, allowing blood to flow more efficiently.

Cardiovascular Exercise Safety Tips

While Wall Pilates offers a gentle way to improve your health, safety is paramount:

Consult your doctor: Before starting any new exercise program, seek clearance from your healthcare provider, especially if you have any preexisting health conditions.

Start slow and progress gradually: Begin with low-intensity exercises and gradually increase the duration and intensity as your fitness level improves.

Listen to your body: Pay close attention to your body's signals. If you experience any pain, discomfort, or dizziness, stop the exercise and consult your doctor.

Stay hydrated: Drink plenty of water before, during, and after your workout to stay hydrated and prevent dehydration.

Warm-up and cool-down: Perform gentle stretches and light movements before and after your workout to prepare your body and prevent injury.

***

Preview of Exercise List

T HIS CHAPTER EQUIPS YOU with various Wall Pilates exercises tailored to improve cardiovascular health and increase energy levels. Consistency is key, so begin slowly and gradually increase frequency and intensity as your fitness level improves. Start your journey with gentle stretches and mindful movements to prepare your body and mind for practice. Then, move on to other stages. These exercises will elevate your heart rate and improve circulation, energising you.

Exercise List

Beginner

Warm-Up (two minutes):

Gentle Neck Rolls: Gently roll your head clockwise and counter-clockwise, feeling the stretch in your neck muscles. Repeat five times in each direction.

Arm Circles: With your arms outstretched at shoulder height, make small circles with your arms forward and backward, gradually increasing the size of the circles. Repeat ten times in each direction.

Wall Marching with Arm Circles:

Stand back against a wall with your feet shoulder-width apart and about an inch away from the wall. Engage your core and maintain good posture with your back straight and shoulders relaxed.

Begin marching in place by lifting your knees to a 90-degree angle with each step. Alternate legs in a steady rhythm.

Simultaneously, start small arm circles in the forward or backward direction (you can alternate directions with each set). Keep your arms extended to the sides at shoulder level.

Focus on coordinating your leg movements with the arm circles, ensuring both motions flow smoothly. Continue marching and circling your arms for 30 seconds to one minute, gradually increasing the intensity as you feel comfortable. Rest for 15-30 seconds and repeat for 2-3 sets.

Wall Jumping Jacks:

Stand facing a wall with your feet hip-width apart and arms at your sides. Jump slightly, raising your arms overhead and spreading your legs apart.

Simultaneously, tap your fingertips on the wall in front of you. Jump back to the starting position, lowering your arms and bringing your legs together.

Repeat for 30-60 seconds at a comfortable pace.

Wall High Knees:

Stand with your back against the wall, your feet hip-width apart. Run in place, bringing your knees high towards your chest with each step.

Maintain a tall posture and keep your core engaged. Repeat for 30-60 seconds at a comfortable pace.

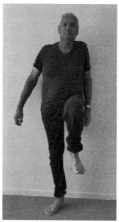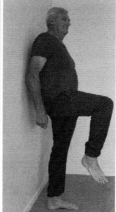

Cool-Down (two minutes):

Deep Breathing: Sit or stand comfortably and take slow, deep breaths through your nose and out your mouth. Repeat for five breaths.

Chest stretch: Clasp your hands behind your back and gently open your chest, pushing your shoulders back.

Intermediate

Warm Up (two minutes): Same as beginner.

Wall Heel Taps:

Stand facing the wall, feet hip-width apart and about an inch away from the wall. Place your hands on the wall for support.

Tap one heel up and down against the wall, keeping your leg straight. Focus on using your ankle muscles to control the movement and maintain a moderate pace. Repeat with the other leg, alternating for two minutes

Wall Leg Swings:

Stand with your side facing a wall with your feet hip-width apart and about an inch away from the wall. Place your hand flat on the wall for balance.

Swing one leg forward and back, keeping your leg straight and core engaged. Avoid using momentum; focus on controlled movements. Repeat 10-15 swings per leg.

Wall Bicycle Crunches:

Lie on your back on the floor with your legs extended and feet against the wall. Place your hands behind your head, elbows out to the sides.

Engage your core and lift your shoulders off the ground, bringing one knee towards your chest while extending the opposite leg straight out. Twist your torso to bring your elbow towards the raised knee.

Alternate sides, mimicking a pedalling motion. Focus on controlled movements and engaging your core throughout the exercise. Repeat ten times on each side.

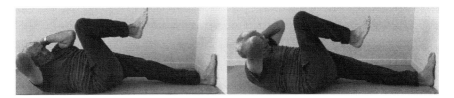

Wall Side Leg Lifts:

Stand beside a wall with your right side towards it. Place your right hand flat on the wall for balance.

Lift your left leg straight to the side, keeping your leg parallel to the floor. Lower your leg back down slowly and with control. Repeat 10-15 repetitions per leg.

Cool Down (two minutes): Same as beginner.

Advanced

Warm Up (two minutes): Same as beginner.

Wall Marching in Place:

Stand with your back against a wall with your feet shoulder-width apart. March in place, bringing your knees high towards your chest at a 90-degree angle.

Keep your back straight and core engaged. Maintain a steady pace for 30-60 seconds.

Wall Arm Raises:

Stand facing a wall with your feet hip-width apart. Place your hands flat on the wall at shoulder height, fingers pointing upwards.

Slowly raise your arms overhead, pressing your palms firmly into the wall. Lower your arms back down to the starting position with control. Repeat 10-15 repetitions.

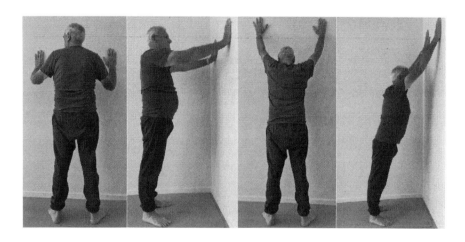

Wall Toe Taps:

Stand facing a wall with your feet hip-width apart and about an inch away from the wall. Standing on your heels, quickly tap your toes against the wall, alternating feet.

Keep your core engaged and maintain a balanced posture. Continue for 30-60 seconds at a fast pace.

Cool Down (two minutes): Same as beginner.

7 DAY FITNESS PROGRAM

Welcome to your 7-Day Workout Program. Let's embrace each day as a new opportunity to grow stronger in body and spirit. The journey of a thousand miles begins with a single step – let your first step be towards the wall, ready to conquer your goals one day at a time.

This program is designed to help you see results within 7 days, it starts with 10 minutes per day and gradually builds up to 15 minutes. The gentle exercises focus on improving strength, flexibility and balance safely. Adjust the exercises as needed to match your fitness level and comfort. Always listen to your body and consult with a healthcare professional before starting any new exercise program.

Day 1: Introduction and Gentle Warm-Up (10 minutes)

Warm-Up (2 minutes)

- **Shoulder Rolls:** Gently roll your head clockwise and counterclockwise, feeling the stretch in your neck muscles. Repeat five times in each direction for a minute.

- **Arm circles:** With your arms outstretched at shoulder height, move your arms forward and backward, making small circles. Slowly increase the size of the circles. Repeat five times in each direction for a minute.

Wall Pilates Exercises (6 minutes)

- **Wall Plank:** Stand facing the wall, place your hands on the wall at shoulder height, and step back until your body forms a straight line. Hold the position for 30 seconds – one minute or as long as you feel comfortable.

- **Wall Squat:** Stand with your back against the wall, feet shoulder-width apart. Slide down the wall into a squat position, engage your core and keep your back straight, hold for 10 seconds, then slide back up. Repeat 10 – 15 times.

- **Wall Arm Raises:** Stand facing a wall with your feet hip-width apart. Place your hands on the wall at shoulder height, fingers pointing upwards. Slowly raise your arms overhead, pressing your palms firmly into the wall. Lower your arms back down to the starting position with control. Repeat 5 – 10 times.

- **Wall Leg Lift:** Lie on your back with your legs bent and feet flat on the floor. Press your lower back into the mat and lift one leg straight up towards the ceiling, keeping your core engaged. Slowly lower the leg back down and repeat with the other leg. Do 10-15 lifts per leg.

Cool Down (2 minutes)

- **Gentle Stretching:** 2 minutes

Day 2: Core and Stability (10 minutes)

Warm-Up (2 minutes)

- **Marching in Place:** Lift your knees high while marching on the spot for one minute.

- **Gentle Side Bends:** Stand with feet shoulder-width apart. Gently bend to one side, reaching your arm over your head, then repeat on the other side for one minute.

Wall Pilates Exercises (6 minutes)

- **Wall Roll Down:** Stand with your back against the wall. Slowly roll down to touch your toes, then roll back up. Repeat 5-10 times.

- **Wall Push-Up:** Stand facing the wall, place your hands on the wall at shoulder height, and perform push-ups for 30 seconds – one minute.

- **Wall Bridge:** Lie on your back with your feet against the wall. Lift your hips to form a bridge, hold for 10 seconds, and lower back down. Repeat for 30 seconds – one minute.

- **Wall Side Leg Raise:** Stand sideways to the wall for support. Lift your outer leg to the side, hold it for 10 seconds and lower it back down. Switch legs and repeat on the other side. Repeat on each leg for 10 – 15 lifts.

Cool Down (2 minutes)

- **Gentle Core Stretches:** 2 minutes

Day 3: Flexibility and Range of Motion (10 minutes)

Warm-Up (2 minutes)

- **Gentle Arm Swings:** Stand with your back to a wall, feet shoulder-width apart, and slightly away from the wall. Slowly swing your arms forward and upward in a controlled motion, aiming to bring them to shoulder height or slightly above. Then, gently swing your arms back down to the starting position. Continue for one minute.

- **Leg Swings:** Place a hand on the wall for stability, and swing one leg forward and backward 10-15 times then repeat on the other leg.

Wall Pilates Exercises (6 minutes)

- **Wall Calf Stretch:** Place your hands on the wall, step one foot back, and press the heel down to stretch the calf. Hold each stretch for 30 seconds. Repeat on both legs twice.

- **Wall Hamstring Stretch:** Place one foot against the wall and gently lean forward to stretch the hamstring. Hold each stretch for 30 seconds. Repeat on both legs once on each side.

- **Wall Chest Opener:** Stand facing the wall, place your hands on the wall and lean forward to open up the chest. Hold for 30 seconds – one minute.

- **Wall Hip Flexor Stretch:** Stand facing the wall with feet hip-width apart. Lean back and place hands shoulder-height on the wall for support. Lift one leg slightly and gently pull your knee towards your chest, feeling a stretch in the front of your thigh and hip. Hold for 30 seconds each leg.

Cool Down (2 minutes)

- **Deep Breathing and Relaxation:** 3 minutes

Day 4: Strength and Conditioning (12 minutes)

Warm-Up (3 minutes)

- **Gentle Walking in Place:** Walk gently around the room, lifting your feet slightly for 1.5 minutes to warm up your body.

- **Shoulder shrugs:** Lift your shoulders towards your ears and then lower them back down for 1.5 minutes.

Wall Pilates Exercises (7 minutes)

- **Wall Chair Pose:** Stand with your back against the wall, slide down into a chair pose, hold for 20 – 30 seconds, and stand back up. Repeat four times.

- **Wall Arm Circles:** Stand facing the wall, extend your arms, and make small circles for two minutes.

- **Wall Toe Tap:** Stand with your back on the wall with your feet hip-width apart and arms down by your sides. Keep your core engaged and back straight. Tap your right heel up and down against the wall, maintaining constant contact. Do 15-20 taps, then switch legs and repeat for three minutes.

Cool Down (2 minutes)

- **Gentle Stretches:** 2 minutes

Day 5: Rest and Recovery (10 minutes)

Gentle Activity

- **Relaxed Walking:** 5 minutes. Walk at a relaxed pace in a comfortable setting.

- **Light Stretching:** 5 minutes. Perform gentle stretches for the whole body.

Day 6: Balance and Coordination (12 minutes)

Warm-Up (2 minutes)

- **Gentle Leg Swings:** Swing each leg forward and backward for 30 seconds with a hand on the wall for stability then switch legs.

- **Arm Circles:** Stand facing the wall, extend your arms, and make small circles for 1 minute.

Wall Pilates Exercises (8 minutes)

- **Wall Standing March:** Stand facing the wall, lift one knee to hip height, then switch legs. Repeat for two minutes.

- **Wall Heel Raise:** Stand facing the wall, rise onto your toes, hold for 20 – 30 seconds, and lower. Repeat for two minutes.

- **Wall Figure-8:** Stand facing the wall, extend your arms, and draw figure-8s with your hands for one to two minutes.

- **Wall Jumping Jacks:** Stand facing a wall with your feet hip-width apart and arms at your sides do jumping jacks for one to two minutes at a comfortable pace.

Cool Down (2 minutes)

- **Gentle Leg and Arm Stretches:** 2 minutes

Day 7: Full Body Integration (15 minutes)

Warm-Up (5 minutes)

- **Gentle Jogging in Place:** Jog in place gently, lifting your feet slightly for 2.5 minutes.

- **Arm Swings:** Perform gentle stretches for the entire body for 2.5 minutes.

Wall Pilates Exercises (8 minutes)

- **Wall Push-Up:** Stand facing the wall, place your hands on the wall at shoulder height, and perform push-ups for 30 seconds – one minute.

- **Wall Squat:** Stand with your back against the wall, feet shoulder-width apart. Slide down the wall into a squat position, engage your core and keep your back straight, hold for 10 seconds, then slide back up. Repeat

10 – 15 times.

- **Wall Roll Down:** Stand with your back against the wall. Slowly roll down to touch your toes, then roll back up. Repeat 5-10 times.

- **Wall Side Leg Raise:** Stand sideways to the wall for support. Lift your outer leg to the side, hold it for 10 seconds and lower it back down. Switch legs and repeat on the other side. Repeat on each leg for 10 – 15 lifts.

Cool Down (2 minutes)

- **Gentle Full Body Stretch:** 2 minutes

Congratulations on completing the 7-Day Wall Pilates for Seniors Challenge! Your dedication and effort have truly paid off. You've taken an important step towards better health and fitness, and your commitment is an inspiration. Keep up the great work, and remember, every day is an opportunity for a stronger, healthier you. Well done!

Now you've mastered the 7-Day Program, move on to the next chapter – the 28-Day Program.

28 DAY FITNESS PROGRAM

Welcome to your 28-Day Workout Program, commit to 28 days of transformation, where each session brings you closer to your best self. Remember, progress is built one step at a time. Embrace the challenge, celebrate the small victories, and believe in the strength within you. This is your journey to a healthier, stronger, and more empowered you.

The program starts with 10 minutes a day and gradually builds up to 15 minutes per day. The gentle exercises focus on improving strength, flexibility and balance safely. Adjust the exercises as needed to match your fitness level and comfort. Always listen to your body and consult with a healthcare professional before starting any new exercise program.

Warm-Up for each day (2 minutes)

- **Shoulder Rolls:** 1 minute

- **Gentle Neck Stretches:** 1 minute

Cool Down for each day (2 minutes)

- **Gentle Stretching:** 2 minutes

Week 1: Introduction (10 minutes/day)

Day 1-2:

1. **Wall Roll Down** - 2 minutes

2. **Wall Squats** - 3 minutes

3. **Wall Arm Circles** - 2 minutes

4. **Wall Push-Ups** - 3 minutes

Day 3:

- Rest Day

Day 4, 5 & 6:

1. **Wall Roll Down** - 2 minutes

2. **Wall Squats** - 3 minutes

3. **Wall Arm Circles** - 2 minutes

4. **Wall Push-Ups** - 3 minutes

Day 7:

- Rest Day

Week 2: Building Strength (10 minutes/day)

Day 8-9:

1. **Wall Roll Down** - 2 minutes

2. **Wall Squats** - 3 minutes

3. **Wall Arm Circles** - 2 minutes

4. **Wall Push-Ups** - 3 minutes

Day 10:

- Rest Day

Day 11, 12 & 13:

1. **Wall Roll Down** - 2 minutes

2. **Wall Squats** - 3 minutes

3. **Wall Arm Circles** - 2 minutes

4. **Wall Push-Ups** - 3 minutes

Day 14:

- Rest Day

Week 3: Adding Variety (12 minutes/day)

Day 15-16:

1. **Wall Roll Down** - 2 minutes

2. **Wall Squats** - 3 minutes

3. **Wall Arm Circles** - 2 minutes

4. **Wall Push-Ups** - 3 minutes

5. **Wall Leg Lifts** - 2 minutes

Day 17:

- Rest Day

Day 18, 19 & 20:

    1. **Wall Roll Down** - 2 minutes

    2. **Wall Squats** - 3 minutes

    3. **Wall Arm Circles** - 2 minutes

    4. **Wall Push-Ups** - 3 minutes

    5. **Wall Leg Lifts** - 2 minutes

Day 21:

- Rest Day

Week 4: Building Endurance (15 minutes/day)

Day 22-23:

    1. **Wall Roll Down** - 2 minutes

    2. **Wall Squats** - 2 minutes

    3. **Wall Arm Circles** - 2 minutes

    4. **Wall Push-Ups** - 4 minutes

    5. **Wall Leg Lifts** - 2 minutes

    6. **Wall Calf Raises** - 3 minutes

Day 24:

- Rest Day

Day 25, 26 & 27:

    1. **Wall Roll Down** - 2 minutes

2. **Wall Squats** - 3 minutes

3. **Wall Arm Circles** - 2 minutes

4. **Wall Push-Ups** - 3 minutes

5. **Wall Leg Lifts** - 2 minutes

6. **Wall Calf Raises** - 3 minutes

Day 28:

* Rest Day

Exercise Descriptions

1. **Wall Roll Down:** Stand with your back against the wall, feet hip-width apart. Slowly roll down one vertebra at a time, keeping your back in contact with the wall. Roll back up slowly.

2. **Wall Squats:** Stand with your back against the wall, feet shoulder-width apart. Slide down into a squat position, ensuring your knees do not go past your toes. Hold for a few seconds and slide back up.

3. **Wall Arm Circles:** Stand with your back against the wall and arms extended out to the sides. Make small circles with your arms, gradually increasing the size of the circles.

4. **Wall Push-Ups:** Stand facing the wall, and place your hands on the wall at shoulder height. Bend your elbows to bring your chest towards the wall, then push back to the starting position.

5. **Wall Leg Lifts:** Stand with your side to the wall, and use the wall for support. Lift one leg to the side and lower it back down. Repeat on the other side.

6. **Wall Calf Raises:** Stand facing the wall and place your hands on the

wall for support. Raise your heels off the ground, then lower them back down.

Congratulations on completing the 28-Day Wall Pilates for Seniors Challenge! Your dedication and perseverance have led you to this incredible achievement. You've shown a remarkable commitment to your health and fitness, and your hard work has truly paid off. Celebrate this milestone and carry forward the strength and confidence you've gained. Well done!

CONCLUSION

THE END OF THE ROUTINE, THE START OF A LIFESTYLE

You have made it to this concluding chapter; congratulations on completing this journey into the world of Wall Pilates! You've learned about the numerous benefits that Wall Pilates offers, like making you more flexible and robust and improving your stance, balance, and even heart health. In addition to these physical benefits, Wall Pilates also has the potential to transform your mental focus, stress levels, and quality of life as a whole.

You now know that Wall Pilates is more than just a set of movements; it's a way of life that can improve every part of your life. Add Wall Pilates to your daily routine, and you'll improve your physical, mental, and emotional health.

Mindfulness is an integral part of Wall Pilates. It means being in the present moment and aware of your body and actions. You can use mindfulness in your daily life and your Wall Pilates exercise to help you stay focused, calm, and centred when life gets tough.

Looking back, consider how far you've come. You've learned:

The power of gentle yet effective movement: Wall Pilates exercises, designed specifically for seniors, have allowed you to improve your flexibility, balance, and strength, all while minimising stress on your joints.

Improved Mobility and Flexibility: You've learned how gentle stretches and exercises can combat stiffness and enhance your range of motion, allowing you to move more easily and confidently in your daily activities.

Reduced Stress and Anxiety: By incorporating mindful movements and breathing techniques, you've discovered how Wall Pilates promotes relaxation, lowers stress hormones, and contributes to a sense of inner peace and well-being.

Enhanced Sleep Quality: By addressing underlying stressors and promoting relaxation, Wall Pilates has equipped you with tools to improve your sleep quality, leaving you feeling refreshed and energised throughout the day.

Improved Cardiovascular Health: You've learned how gentle, low-impact exercises and mindful breathing can strengthen your heart, increase your stamina, and contribute to a healthier cardiovascular system.

The benefits of breathing techniques: Diaphragmatic breathing, a cornerstone of Wall Pilates, empowers you to better manage stress, improve circulation, and enhance your overall health.

These among others. And remember, this is just the beginning. The beauty of Wall Pilates lies in its versatility and adaptability. As you continue your practice, you can:

Explore new exercises: Each week, you can gradually incorporate more challenging exercises or variations to challenge your body and mind continuously.

Focus on specific goals: Whether you want to improve your balance for everyday activities, increase your stamina, or maintain your current fitness level, Wall Pilates offers endless possibilities to tailor your practice to your individual needs.

Embark on a lifelong journey: Wall Pilates transcends mere exercise; it embodies a lifestyle fostering physical and mental wellness. Dedicate yourself to consistent participation, and observe as it seamlessly integrates into your daily regimen, enriching your life for the long term.

Wall Pilates is beneficial because it can be changed to fit different needs and goals, whether you're a beginner who wants to get in better shape or an expert practitioner who wants to try something new. The exercises are easy but still work, making them suitable for people of all ages and fitness levels.

There are many great testimonies on the vast benefits of wall pilates. I have witnessed and experienced these benefits myself, and I can tell you that it's a journey that will distinguish you from others and leave you without regrets.

Always pay attention to your body and do what it needs as you move through Wall Pilates. Take it easy when you need to, and push yourself when ready. Your strength, flexibility, and general health will improve with your practice.

Remember that Wall Pilates is more than just working out; it's about caring for your body, mind, and spirit. Accept the power of Wall Pilates and see how it changes your body and life.

Thank you for joining me on this journey. May your practice of Wall Pilates bring you joy, vitality, and peace.

MAKE A DIFFERENCE WITH YOUR REVIEW

Now you have everything you need to reclaim your vitality and redefine your later years; it's time to pass on your newfound knowledge and show other readers where they can find the same help.

Simply by leaving your honest opinion of this book on Amazon, you'll show other seniors where they can find the information they're looking for and promote their passion for staying active and healthy.

I appreciate your help. The journey to better health and vitality is kept alive when we pass on our knowledge – and you're helping us to do just that

Your review can make a difference for someone who's on the fence about starting their journey into wall pilates. Share your thoughts and tell them how this book has impacted your life.

Remember, your experiences and insights can be the guiding light for others seeking the benefits of wall pilates.

Thank you once again for being a part of this journey and for sharing the love of wall pilates with others.

Your biggest fan, Laurel Harris

Scan the QR code to leave your review!

OTHER BOOKS IN THE SERIES

Thank you so much for joining me on this journey through Chair Yoga & Wall Pilates for Seniors.

If you are interested in any other books in the Fitness and Self Help for Seniors Series please check out my other books below – thank you.

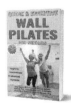

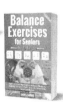
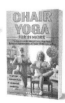

REFERENCES

ACE Fitness, (n.d.). 5 Benefits of Flexibility Training. online Available at: https://www.acefitness.org/resources/everyone/blog/6646/benefits-of-flexibility/.

BetterMe, (n.d.). Wall Pilates For Beginners: 8 Effective Exercises To Strengthen Your Core And Tone Your Muscles. online Available at: https://betterme.world/articles/wall-pilates-for-beginners.

Bustle, (n.d.). 6 Beginner Wall Pilates Exercises That Will Seriously Work Your Core. online Available at: https://www.bustle.com/wellness/beginner-wall-pilates-exercises.

Harvard Health Publishing, (n.d.). The benefits of flexibility exercises. online Available at: https://www.health.harvard.edu/staying-healthy/benefits-of-flexibility-exercises.

Livestrong, (n.d.). A Wall Pilates Workout That'll Help You Get a Full-Body Workout Without Any Equipment. online Available at: https://www.livestrong.com/article/13776995-wall-pilates-workout.

Mayo Clinic, (n.d.). Stretching: Focus on flexibility. online Available at: https://www.mayoclinic.org/healthy-lifestyle/fitness/in-depth/stretching/art-20047931.

Today, (n.d.). Wall Pilates: The Fast Fitness Trend People Are Raving About. online Available at: https://www.today.com/health/diet-fitness/wall-pilates-exercises-rcna103846.

Verywell Fit, (n.d.). 10 Basic Pilates Moves for Beginners. online Available at: https://www.verywellfit.com/exercises-for-pilates-beginners-2704717.

Verywell Health, (n.d.). The Importance of Flexibility and How to Improve It. online Available at: https://www.verywellhealth.com/why-is-flexibility-important-7567252.

Women's Health, (n.d.). 20-Minute Pilates Workout for Beginners. online Available at: https://www.womenshealthmag.com/fitness/g44077939/pilates-for-beginners-workout-video/.